MICHAEL ALEXANDER is the pseudonym of a nurse who has previously worked in the UK and New Zealand.

Also by Michael Alexander

Confessions of a Male Nurse
Getting Out Alive (ebook)

MICHAEL ALEXANDER

Confessions of a
School Nurse

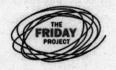

The Friday Project
An imprint of HarperCollins*Publishers*
1 London Bridge Street
London SE1 9GF

www.harpercollins.co.uk

This edition published by The Friday Project in 2015

ISBN: 978-0-00-758642-4

Printed and bound in England by
Clays Ltd, St Ives plc

MIX
Paper from
responsible sources
FSC **FSC® C007454**
www.fsc.org

FSC™ is a non-profit international organisation established to promote
the responsible management of the world's forests. Products carrying the
FSC label are independently certified to assure consumers that they come
from forests that are managed to meet the social, economic and
ecological needs of present and future generations,
and other controlled sources.

Find out more about HarperCollins and the environment at
www.harpercollins.co.uk/green

To Mum and Dad

Disclaimer

The stories described in this book are based on my experiences working as a school nurse in boarding schools over the past ten years. To protect confidentiality, some parts are fictionalised and all places and names are changed, but nonetheless they remain an honest reflection of the variety and crazy goings-on witnessed during a decade's worth of school nursing – surprising as that might come to seem!

CONTENTS

PROLOGUE

A Taste

Marcus made sure no one was sitting near the door before closing it.

'It's really personal,' he whispered to me over his shoulder.

'It has to be a guy,' he'd insisted when he arrived at the bustling nurses' office. Most requests of this nature are girls asking to see a female nurse; though this was only my first week in the role, Marcus was the first student to ask to see a man, so my mind went into overdrive imagining the ways in which I could impart my knowledge in a reassuring, helpful manner to a young man in obvious need.

As Marcus turned from the door to face me, his hands delved into the front of his pants. He wasn't in uniform; he wore loose track pants instead. I got the feeling than an inspection of that area was on the horizon. He refused a seat, so I asked him what the problem was.

'You won't tell anyone?' he answered.

'Of course I won't tell anyone, just explain what's wrong.'

'They're sore. My nuts are sore. And the left one seems bigger.'

Ah!

I could either take a look at Marcus now, or wait for him to be seen at the local doctor's office. I chose the latter. There was no need for the poor lad to be exposing himself more than necessary. It's not that Dr Fritz wouldn't have trusted my judgment, but there's more to feeling someone's nuts than the average guy thinks. Is there a lump? Does it move freely? Is it attached to the testicle? Is the spermatic cord twisted? It would be up to Dr Fritz to decide what to do – whether it would require an urgent scan today or was something that could wait – so he would need to examine the lad properly. And besides, this environment wasn't ideal for an intimate examination; the south wall of my office was made of glass, a window that looked out upon the mountains and a large terrace … a window with no curtain.

But Marcus was too quick for me.

'You have to see them,' he declared, whipping his pants down. Looking up, he gave a short scream.

No students were on the terrace, but Mrs Driscoll, the head-master's wife, was there with what looked like a prospective family … admiring the view.

Despite the incident, the prospective girl did enroll. Rumour has it she insisted.

Now don't worry, I'll get back to Marcus's nuts in a minute, but before I do, let me tell you how I came to be here on this snowy mountain.

The first day

Why did I become a school nurse?

At the age of 32, I was a skilled professional with more than ten years' experience working in England and New Zealand. I was a highly trained emergency specialist, who had worked in some of the biggest hospitals and busiest departments in the world, and the money wasn't too bad. Why would I leave all of that? At that time, school nursing didn't even seem like real nursing to me.

But, I needed a healthier lifestyle. Thirty pounds an hour sounds great at first, but the irregular night shifts – one on, one off, two on then one off – it ruins you. That's what temp or agency nursing is about in London; you take the work when you can, even if that means spending your weekends with a bunch of drunks, dealing with abuse and violence, as well as the two-hour commute to and from the hospital. I'd chosen that life, but it's not doable long term, and besides, there was a much bigger factor at play. My partner and I were expecting our first child, and I wanted a safe, healthy environment in which to raise my family.

My choice seemed simple, go back to my homeland, New Zealand, and get my old job back, or find work somewhere in Europe that had regular hours, no drunks, no night shifts, no underground and clean air. I didn't feel that going back to New Zealand to work in a regular ward or a small emergency department was right for me, especially as my partner had never even been to my hometown, and we both wanted to stay close to her family for our first child.

So when I saw an advert for a nurse to work at a boarding school in the Alps, I thought all my wishes had come true. It not only seemed to fit all my requirements, they also even offered me a chalet in the middle of a ski resort. What more could a nurse with half a dozen ski seasons behind him ask for?

I applied and after a phone interview, background and police check (I'd be living and working with children, after all) I was offered the job.

Walking into my new office on that first day with Mr Driscoll, the headmaster, made me forget about big city life almost immediately.

The southern wall of the school consisted of a window looking out onto towering peaks over 3000 metres, the highest already capped with snow, despite only being late August. I felt a pang of guilt thinking the view was even better than what I was used to back in New Zealand.

Yes. I knew I'd made the right decision for me and my budding family. I felt this could be home.

'You're free to do as you see fit,' Mr Driscoll said as he showed us around the clinic. My colleagues in crime, Justine and Michaela, glanced at me in surprise. None of us had ever worked in a boarding school before; we had all come from the frontline of the nursing profession, used to being surrounded by large teams. We had taken the leap from the Accident and Emergency to an elite boarding school. We had a clean slate.

Justine was from Alaska. She had spent the last ten years in emergency medicine and had come over with her husband who had a job as a maths teacher at the school.

Michaela was from Minneapolis and specialised in paediatric emergency medicine. She had also come with her husband; they had always wanted to live in Europe.

'With your combined experience, I trust you'll do a great job,' Mr Driscoll added. And with that, he left us to it. The school was to be our playground.

On our first day at work, we found out that we were alone; alone and in charge of 400 students, some of the world's most privileged children. There was no on-site doctor lurking in the background who we could turn to for help; no alarm button to press when things turned sour; no oxygen, no intravenous access, none of the equipment that I'd gotten used to having on hand, ready for instant use.

The 400 children came from over fifty nationalities, and while the majority spoke English to a high standard at least ten per cent knew little or none of the language. Other than English, the next most common tongue was Russian.

The other nurses and I were to be responsible for keeping the children healthy, taking care of them when they were ill or hurt, helping them to get along with each other, counselling them through life's hurdles, and arming them with the knowledge that comes from being an 'old woman' or 'old man' who has made it this far in life without too many major screw-ups (the fact that we're not even grey doesn't seem to matter to the kids).

I was looking forward to the challenge. No longer would I have to deal with shootings, stabbings, heart attacks, strokes, violent drunks or demented, incontinent or suicidal patients. Instead, I was going to be looking after fit, young, healthy teenagers. How hard could that be?

The parents had spent a fortune to send their kids here: 100,000 euros per child per year. I assumed they would be hardworking, motivated, intelligent, considerate, good-natured, balanced individuals …

However, as you'll discover over the course of this book, I'm not always great with assumptions.

Marcus's jewels

'Why didn't you tell me?' Marcus cried, whipping up his tracksuit bottoms to hide himself from the family crowd gathered outside.

I bundled Marcus out the office, into the car and off to the local doctor's office. Thankfully, Dr Fritz's surgery is in the centre of the village, only a five-minute drive away.

Proximity and willingness alone made Dr Fritz the unofficial school doctor. In addition to running a full-time GP practice, he was also our first port of call if there was an issue the nursing staff felt needed a doctor's opinion, and we would make an appointment at his office and send the child along. Even on his time off, it was not uncommon for him to see our students if the matter was urgent. Dr Fritz was also there if a student needed specialist help, as he knew who the closest and best experts were, and referrals were made through him.

Like all born and bred mountain men, Dr Fritz is a no-nonsense man. He's also one of the hardest working GPs I've ever met. He is always there during the day or available in the middle of the night, no matter what, and it wasn't unusual for him to put in an eighty-hour week.

He even has the 'unique quirks' that often come not only with living in an isolated mountain village, but being the only GP for a whole community.

He was happy to see Marcus straight away. Pain in the testicles can be very serious. Torsion (a twisted spermatic cord) is a surgical emergency. Within minutes, the doctor had Marcus lying on the examination table.

He began his assessment as all doctors do, by examining the whole person and not just the affected part, and gradually worked his way to Marcus's testicles. I had wondered if he was going to glove-up as he doesn't always, and in this case didn't, although he was completely professional in his exam. At one point Marcus raised an eyebrow and gave me a worried look, but he kept quiet. It isn't wise to question any man who has your nuts resting in the palm of their bare hands.

Once the examination was over, Dr Fritz arranged for an ultrasound scan to take place as soon as possible.

'I do not think it is a torsion,' he explained, 'but we need to be sure.' We were standing by the reception desk, as he turned the pages of his diary. He licked the index finger of his right hand to turn another page … the same hand he'd just used to feel Marcus's testicles.

I glanced at Marcus to see if he had noticed, and saw him staring at the doctor's hand, his mouth hanging open. He leant towards me and whispered in an appalled tone, 'He just tasted my balls.'

Dr Fritz does wear gloves when strictly necessary, has always been proper and he did wash his hands, but not before the ultrasound had been arranged. Where other doctors usually wear gloves when examining warts, fungusy toes, and the like, Dr Fritz doesn't. I don't agree with Dr Fritz sometimes, but he is completely trustworthy if a little unprofessional – you wouldn't get away with it in most places, and in a way, that shows just how unique this little community is.

This was the first of many peculiarities I would eventually come across while working with the doctor.

As for Marcus, the ultrasound showed that he had a hydrocele, or a little cyst full of fluid, attached to his left testicle, that is absolutely harmless. Marcus calmed down a great deal once he realised his balls weren't going to drop off, and the pain settled with some ibuprofen.

As first weeks go, this was pretty ridiculous … but, as I was to find out, this was just the beginning.

CHAPTER ONE

The Transition

Luke

I have a confession to make: before seeing the school vacancy, I had never planned on working with children. But I figured it wouldn't be too hard. I'd learned some of the general rules during my years in the emergency room; developed the hunches that seep into the core of any nurse or doctor who spends their life looking after others.

A screaming child is a good thing, although not for one's ears. It means a set of functioning lungs and an airway that is clear. A child that fights as you struggle to put in an IV or suck some blood is also a good sign, it means their illness hasn't sapped too much of their life force. A child that is quiet, a child that doesn't put up a fight, is a concern. Their illness has begun to overthrow their natural survival instincts.

Luke was quiet. He was nine years old and one of the youngest children at our school. He was also one of my earliest patients.

The junior school consists of about sixty children, an almost even split of boys and girls from ages 9–12, and while they do sometimes mingle with the high school kids, they live and study separately. They do, however, share the same nurse. I see the little ones and the big ones.

'What's wrong?' I asked as I ushered a pale, sunken Luke into the examination room. He mumbled a reply and I asked him to speak a little louder.

'I feel sick,' he managed, his chin resting on his chest, his eyes staring blankly at the ground.

The words 'I'm sick' don't really help a lot, but he wasn't up to giving me a more useful answer. To investigate, I phoned up the people in charge of his dorm to get a bit of background.

'He's had a bit of a cough,' Mrs Pierce his dorm parent explained. 'I didn't realise he was so sick. He was running around with the others playing football this morning. I'm so sorry.'

The people in charge of the dorms are usually a married couple of any age, but often with their own children, and they're the heart of all boarding schools, wherever they may be. They act as a parent to these children, hence the title.

Mrs Pierce sounded defensive, but she had no need to be. Kids are renowned for bouncing off the walls one minute, then being deathly sick the next. They reach that tipping point where their reserves are finally exhausted and their body suddenly catches onto the idea that it's unwell.

With Luke I, at least, had a starting point – a cough and a runny nose. He also had a high temperature, 39.9. I was worried, not because of his illness, but because it was up to me to make the call on what to do. I could make the five-minute drive to the doctor's office, but Dr Fritz is a busy man. He has a whole village to take care of, and I can't go running to him every time a child has a high fever. To help me decide, I did what I would do if triaging someone in the emergency room. I got as much data as possible.

No headache, no neck stiffness, no rash and no photophobia (sensitivity to light) plus a probable cause for his fever, that is, a cough and runny nose; probably a simple cold.

Lungs clear, with good air entry on both sides with no wheezes, crackles or signs of respiratory distress and his pulse and blood pressure were fine. But he oozed misery. His body ached and shivered. 'I'm so cold,' he mumbled.

It's normal to feel cold when your temperature is up. Sometimes it's the first sign you notice when someone is sick; you'll find them nestled under two duvets with a hot water bottle, trying to warm up, and when you check their temperature, it's very high.

'You're going to stay with us for a bit,' I explained as I led him through to the sick bay. We have sixteen beds for 400 kids. The most sick get the beds, while the not so sick stay in their dorm where their dorm parent takes care of them. Luke probably had a simple cold, but such a high temperature needed to be monitored.

'Please don't take it away!' Luke screamed, horrified that I'd removed the duvet and replaced it with a thin blanket. It was the most he'd reacted since being admitted. It's cruel, watching him shiver, and it didn't help when I placed a cool compress on his forehead. But he was only nine years old and did as told.

Over the next couple of hours, the combination of cooling measures, paracetamol and half a litre of water brought his temperature back down to 37.2, and his actions showed.

'Can I watch a movie?' is a sign that a child is getting better. I set him up with something to watch. Once the movie was over, this was followed by 'I'm bored'. I love those words. They're almost as good as 'I'm hungry'. Sure signs of recovery.

All the same, I kept Luke in the health centre that night. Illness comes in waves, and Luke didn't disappoint. His temperature went up and down, dragging his body along for the ride, but by the following morning he was feeling good again, and after a day with no fever or body aches, he was sent back to his dorm.

Why had I been so worried? Why had I even considered sending him to the doctor? I knew he had a simple cold, and I know that children are adept at taking onboard very high fevers.

It was because I was the one making the ultimate decision, although it did help having two experienced colleagues to turn to. But I was the one making the decisions, especially late at night or on the weekend, and deciding if a fever was benign, or a sign of something more sinister, even life threatening, and I was the one going to sleep at night wondering 'what if?'. There were no doctors in the background to run a reassuring eye over him, and no blood tests to see how his white blood cells were holding the fort, or inflammatory markers to see how much of a battering his body was taking. I was using my senses and basic observations to make what seemed like a simple call.

But nothing is simple, and in medicine, the simplest decisions don't happen without a lot of thought. This is my job now. I'm the decision maker, the responsible one. It's terrifying.

Learning the basics

'*Shit*,' I thought to myself as yet another girl burst into tears. That was three already this morning. What the hell was I doing? Am I some sort of monster?

No, I was just doing what I had done for the last half dozen years – triaging the students as if this were an A&E department.

'My nose is blocked,' said Marie. I handed her a box of tissues and moved on to the next patient.

'I feel dizzy,' said Sarah. Blood pressure fine, pulse steady and strong, no medical history of note, but skipped breakfast – treated with banana and told to return to class.

'I've got a cough,' said Isabelle. Chest clear, cough non-productive, dry, had only for 24 hours, no fever, otherwise well, and has not coughed once in the last thirty minutes she's been in the waiting room – told to take some cough syrup if it comes back, no treatment at present.

Marie hadn't made it out to the hallway before the flood of tears began again. I stood and watched helplessly as she sat back down between Sarah and Isabelle, who instantly put their arms around her. For teenage girls, tears are contagious, and within moments the three of them were weeping quietly, hands entwined, consoling each other with mumbled words and the occasional glance in my direction, pleading with their eyes for some sign of compassion from me.

I'd never managed to upset three fourteen-year-old girls at once before, but I was doing a fine job of it. I'd even made it an international event, as Marie was Italian, Sarah American, and Isabelle from Russia. I'd covered half the globe.

What the heck should I do?

I did what any male would do when confronted with such a convincing scene. I ran for the hills!

Not really.

I let all three of them rest in the bedroom for an hour and made them some camomile tea with honey.

'We won't bother you again all week,' promised Marie as she went back to class.

'Thank you so much,' said Sarah.

'You didn't forget to excuse us from class?' asked Isabelle, making sure they didn't get an absence marked on the computer.

'You're all excused. No need to worry,' I assured them.

I had just let myself be played. They knew it, and they also knew I knew they knew. I suspect they felt obliged to push the limits. They had three new nurses, completely new to the world of boarding schools, and in these first few months everyone was still figuring out their boundaries. But if I was to continue treating these students like we were in a hospital trauma centre, I was never going to come out on top. I had to come up with another strategy, because if 90 per cent of the patients I had seen this morning had turned up to their local hospital, they would have been encouraged to turn away, or put at the back of the queue and wait hours to be seen.

Hospitals are great for treating accidents and the seriously unwell, but my role as a boarding school nurse was much more than just looking after the sick.

I'm more than a nurse; I'm a parent to these kids, a discipli-narian, an example, a counsellor, a mentor and often a dry shoulder to cry on. It sometimes means playing along with them and their antics, their dramas, and it also means knowing when and how to set limits – you have to know when to say 'enough is enough'.

One moment I can be reprimanding a kid for bad behaviour, the next I'm consoling a child whose grandfather has just died. Before starting this job I had reasoned that my role would be varied and that I would end up doing things outside my job description. What I was not prepared for was to constantly be playing detective.

In a hospital setting, you tend to believe what the patient tells you. This makes sense as most people don't like waiting hours to be seen for no reason. But everything's different in a school, where students are looking for excuses to get out of class or homework.

To avoid being taken advantage of, I began to develop some unique (patent pending) assessment techniques.

'Sir, I've got a sore throat' was one of the most common complaints. After a quick peek at their throat I could usually tell if they were exaggerating, or outright lying. If it looked OK and they had no fever, I would send them to class with some lozenges and paracet-amol. This was never the desired result, and within my second week on the job, the children had become resilient to my tactics.

'I vomited during the night, and my throat is sore,' said Marie, the very same Marie who had burst into tears only a week earlier with a blocked nose. Marie had not kept her promise about staying away, she had already become a regular.

Every year there are a dozen or so regulars who stop by two or three times a week, and the reasons vary. They may be homesick, or it may be their first time being unwell without their mother around. Often this changes once they make friends or figure out where they fit in. Sometimes all they need is a wave, a smile, a nod of the head that says 'I'm here for you' and 'you belong'.

The problem with Marie was that she looked in fantastic health. Sure, she could have been up all night vomiting, and one symptom of a bad sore throat (strep throat) is actually an upset stomach so her history does need to be taken seriously as there are potential complications. However, while this is plausible, generally if the throat looks fine, and they have no fever, then I'm stuck with a healthy looking student, with a normal looking throat, who simply claims they've been up most of the night vomiting.

'Your throat is probably sore because of so much vomiting,' I tentatively suggested, 'and your throat actually looks fine, you're not pale, and your tummy doesn't seem to be making too much noise …' My voice trailed off as Marie looked ready to shed some tears, but I completed the ritual: 750mg paracetamol (based on her weight), throat lozenges, honey and camomile tea, and a late pass to class.

'Can't I rest, for just one class?' she asked, but her heart was no longer in it. She had won a partial victory with a late pass, my kindness and a detailed explanation of what my examination had found – nothing – and she relented and left, although I did offer her a vomit bowl on the way out, telling her to 'come back if you fill it up'.

When they don't get the reaction they want, occasionally a student's mouth drops open, they pull out their iPhones and dial their parents. Others just head to class. Fortunately, this relationship had moved on from that first teary-eyed encounter, and Marie and I had come to an unacknowledged yet mutual understanding, where she got the full works – medicines, honeyed tea and a late pass – and did not cry or insist on resting in bed. She took the bowl with a sheepish smile. She was 'well enough' to appreciate my wry stab at humour.

I'm usually vindicated by lunch break when I see the kids who were supposedly up all night vomiting disregarding my advice about avoiding fried/heavy food, eating fries and hamburgers at lunchtime with no obvious ill effects.

Of course, I did get it wrong sometimes, and continue to do so even now from time to time, but I was adapting. I'd sussed the kids out – who were the ones to keep an eye on – and in turn they were beginning to work me out too.

Agent trouble

'You will let her rest now,' demanded Mr Kowski. My finger itched closer to the 'end call' button, but I controlled my temper and my ego. Mr Kowski is far from the first, and will definitely not be the last person to have a go at me. The skill is in keeping your voice steady and calm.

Mr Kowski was calling from Moscow and was Irina's agent.

Irina had just turned fifteen, but was already a regular in the first couple of months of school; at least two to three times a week. As far I could tell she had received great care – the camomile tea, late pass to class, the full check-up of subjective symptoms.

She'd come to the health centre this morning at two minutes to eight, right before the bell for morning class.

Irina claimed she was up all night vomiting, and had not slept, and was having to constantly run to the toilet. But I didn't believe her.

Why didn't I believe her?

Everything was normal. Her stomach was quiet, her temperature fine, her pulse and blood pressure normal, her lips and tongue moist, with none of that furry ugliness you normally get when your stomach contents are forced up and out. But people can have normal observations and still be sick. What they don't do is look so great.

Irina's eyes weren't tired, they were lively, and she smelled good, of quality perfume, not the stench of recycled acid and dehydration. She'd also waited until the last minute to see me as well. When you're that sick, you can't wait to get someone to help. I find the genuinely sick waiting for me to open the door at seven in the morning still in their pyjamas.

After an examination I had tried to send her to her lessons, with no success. Instead of tears, she chose a more formidable weapon. She pulled out her iPhone.

Irina's parents were furious, and like many of our students from non-English speaking countries, they had someone else speak on their behalf. Saudi and South American families usually have a secretary, a family friend who takes care of business, while the Eastern European families have agents. They use an intermediary either because their English is not good enough, or because they're too busy to deal with minor issues like a sick child.

The family secretaries tend to be nice, while the agents are rarely so friendly. 'I'm paid to be angry,' one agent even confessed. 'If a parent shouts at me, then I'm to shout at you.' But I wasn't going to ask Mr Kowski if his bravado was just an act.

I'm convinced yelling is a cultural thing. In some places, to yell at those under you, especially if you're the one paying their salary, is normal, and I've even had students admit that if their fathers didn't yell at their employees, nothing would be done. 'They expect it,' they explained.

I told Mr Kowski that, from my medical experience, Irina appeared well. 'Are you saying she's lying?' His tone had quietened, but the threat no less.

'Yes, she's lying,' I wanted to shout. Even good kids try to pull a fast one sometimes.

'I'm not saying she wasn't sick. What I am saying is that physically she seems well, and seems to have made a fantastic recovery.'

'That may be so, but you make her rest, or else.' Some battles are not worth fighting; they'll cost you too much.

Irina spent the morning asleep. She had no further vomiting and I did not see her get up once to go to the bathroom.

I had to find a better way to get to the truth.

To aid me in my quest for certainty, I developed the PMU test. If a female turns up to the clinic in the morning, claiming she has a sore throat and has been up all night vomiting, but her make-up is immaculate and she looks great, then she has failed the Positive Make-Up test, and I am less likely to believe her. Obviously, this test is only applicable to girls.

Take Sara. Sara couldn't see: 'Sir, my eyes, everything is blurry,' she insisted. She actually reached down, feeling for the chair behind her. This was one of the more unusual presentations, but I wasn't concerned. She'd not only navigated her way out of her dorm and into the health centre, but her eye-liner was straight and her mascara not too heavy or too light, but just right. Her eyesight improved dramatically when I volunteered to be her guide and walk her to class. She nearly missed her English test.

Whereas Angela hadn't slept an ounce. 'My diarrhoea has been non-stop.' She limped in with the assistance of her roommate, because that's what diarrhoea does I guess. Both of them had perfect make-up. Obviously the bathroom didn't smell bad enough to keep them away from the mirror, but I kept Angela for one hour during which I saw no symptoms. After forgetting to limp around my office, she made her way back to class having missed her PE class.

I can't remember any patient in my twenty years of nursing putting on make-up after a miserable night spent in the loo emptying the contents of their stomach. I'm not talking about a touch of lippy, or a brush with some colour, I'm talking about the sort of make-up you use when preparing to take on the town, the complete works.

This was a breakthrough: a simple positive or negative test, which would help me sort the real from the fakes.

But unfortunately, it was only a matter of weeks before some of the students figured this out.

I'm not sure how they cottoned on to it, although I suspect Irina was the first to make the connections. A month after my run in with her agent, Irina turned up again with the same stomach problem, but this time without the layers of make-up, no perfume, a nice bedhead of hair, and wearing pyjamas.

Now I was stuck with a healthy looking patient, with no symptoms, no make-up, claiming she had a sore throat and had been up all night vomiting.

'Who are you?' I said when I first saw Irina in such a state. Oddly, without her make-up she actually looked healthier and brighter, more natural.

'Sir, I'm sick, don't make fun of me.'

It was at this stage that I gave up. If a child is so determined not to go to school, my job is not to figure out what is fact or fiction, but to go by their history. So I let her go to bed, but I made sure she had a bowl to throw up in, and told her I expected to see some vomit, or else.

After nearly ten years looking after school children, I've learned to pick the genuine from the not so genuine, but my greatest fear is missing the one child who looks only mildly unwell and sending them on their way with something major. This problem is exacerbated by the fact that on a day when there are activities, such as skiing, hiking or swimming, I can easily see up to fifty kids, all trying to get a medical excuse. Everyone loved such activities in my time, but this generation is different, delicate even.

But back then, I was still finding my feet. I had to rethink my strategy as to how best to manage the children.

Taking the lead

I could no longer just take patients at their word, especially when all their symptoms were so subjective. And I clearly still had a lot to learn.

'I have a migraine.'

'Are you sure?'

'I have a migraine – a headache.'

'There's a difference between a migraine and a headache, do you have any symptoms?'

Chrissy sighed and rolled her eyes as if speaking to a simpleton. 'My … head … is … sore.'

The 'migraine' sufferers are the easiest to catch. A real migraine sufferer looks absolutely miserable, and just wants to lie down with a pillow over their head and a bucket beside them. Not only did Chrissy look fine, she also had the energy to be sarcastic and roll her eyes. But knowing someone's lying doesn't necessarily make it easier to catch them out.

'How do you know it's a migraine?' I asked.

'Mum has them, and she said I do as well.' So many people have no idea of any of the symptoms of a true migraine. But perhaps Chrissy had the beginnings of one.

'Do you feel like vomiting?' She nodded her head.

'Visual disturbance?' Another nod.

'Dizziness?' Of course.

I naïvely asked her to rate her pain on a scale of 1 to 10, with 10 being the worst pain she could ever imagine.

'Nine or ten.'

She seemed prepared to say yes to every symptom I described. She should be curled up on the floor, her arms wrapped over her head, pleading for us to put her out of her misery.

'It sounds like a real bad one, you've probably got some diarrhoea as well.' Chrissy thought over her response, unsure if I was testing her (which I was) before suggesting that things had seemed a little 'looser' than normal that morning. I gave up. Two 500mg tablets of paracetamol, one hour rest, and she went back to class, symptom free. I found out later that she had missed her Maths test because she was resting in the health centre.

What did I learn? I learnt to keep my mouth shut, which is quite different to what I'd do in an emergency room. When you've got a forty-year-old man with chest pain, you question their symptoms because it helps define the problem, and may just save their life. Questions like 'Does the pain go down your left arm?' or 'Do you have pain in the jaw?' are absolutely vital.

But at the school, I didn't want to ask them if they had any visual disturbance, nausea, vomiting, aura, pins and needles, as the moment I gave them some symptoms to choose from, they usually chose the lot. Without fail, those who have real migraines know their symptoms and do not hesitate to let me know.

Basketball

I like Sunday nights at the school, because they're usually pretty quiet nights to be on call. There are no activities, no drinking (that we know of) and usually little chance of the kids getting into trouble because they're back in their dorm preparing for the week.

But when the phone rang at 8pm one Sunday I received a rude awakening.

'You have to come quickly, there's blood everywhere. Come now, quick!'

The line went dead. I was about to press redial when the phone rang again. 'Sorry, it's me, Brian. I'm in the gym; you have to come quickly, Steve's real bad.'

Brian was the coach of the school basketball team. He was normally a level-headed guy, but like many people involved in nasty looking accidents, when the adrenaline kicks in, they're not the most coherent. I told him to slow down, take a couple of deep breaths, and tell me what happened.

After a pause: 'We were playing basketball, practising for the tournament next weekend. Steve took a fall. It's his arm. There's blood everywhere. I don't know what happened; it's real bad.' An arm injury with lots of blood didn't sound good at all. The

21

worst-case scenario I could think of involving bones and blood was a compound fracture, that is, a broken bone that is also poking through the skin.

I could hear screaming in the background and grabbed my first-aid kit and car keys and headed out the door.

I walked into chaos. There were two adults with Steve, and a horde of boys surrounding them all offering advice at the same time. Yet through all this noise I could hear Steve screaming in agony.

I was the only medic on the scene and it was up to me to do the right thing.

'Don't move him.' As I pushed my way through the crowd, the kids were yelling their diagnoses.

'It's his back, he's broke his back.'

'Oh shit, there's blood everywhere, I think I'm gonna puke.'

As I reached Steve and knelt beside him, I grabbed the shoulder of James, the assistant coach, and ordered him to remove all the boys from the gym. Some resisted, determined to help, others were happy to be led into the foyer, speechless, helpless, but grateful for some direction.

In any situation where there's a crowd, the best thing you can do is to have someone remove the onlookers. I've seen a lot of people with what initially appears to be a serious injury calm down and walk away without any problem once the jittery, frenzied bystanders have been removed. It's also impossible to do an assessment with a screaming horde of onlookers.

Steve was sitting on his backside, clutching his right arm, the front of his shirt covered in blood. I breathed a sigh of relief when I realised the blood wasn't coming from an open wound on his arm but from his nose.

I imagined myself back in the triage room. One of the basic rules of triage is the ABC:

A – his airway was clear, although his nose still had a trickle of blood coming from it.

B – judging by the groans of pain his breathing was fine.

And as for his C – well, he hadn't passed out and he was able to sit so he had an adequate circulation.

Clearly something was wrong and causing a lot of pain, but it was probably not life threatening just yet. I asked him what had happened.

'Please just do something … it's killing me.'

I promised Steve I would do something shortly, but stressed that I did need to know what happened.

Steve had been jumping for a shot when he received an elbow to the nose and came down on his right shoulder. He said he hadn't hit his head or lost consciousness.

It's tempting to tackle the most obvious injury first, and while I could see him clutching his arm, I wanted to be doubly sure to rule out any possible head injury and anything more substantial than a bleeding nose. Alongside the A, B, C is an often unknown little addition, another C, for C-spine.

C-spine, in other words, the bones that make up your neck, should always be checked for injury before moving a patient. The problem is, I've only ever assisted the doctors when they do such things. I'm the one who leads the 'log-roll' when turning patients with possible back injuries. I'm the one who holds the neck still while the doctor gently prods his finger around the back of the neck. If I stuff up and make a sudden move, it can mean a patient is paralysed for life. But now it was up to me to decide the best course of action.

'Is your neck sore?' I asked.

'It's my arm, please just fix the bloody arm, please do something,' he begged. But I didn't get a definitive 'yes' or 'no', and I had to be sure.

'I'm sorry mate, I'll get to the arm next, but I have to know for sure. Were you knocked out at all, and is the back of your head or neck sore?'

'Geez, they're fine, the arm, please …'

To be 100 per cent confident, I placed my fingers on the back of his neck and he denied feeling any pain when I gently pushed. I moved on to the arm.

I asked Steve to sit up straight and he tried, but he wouldn't let go of his right arm. 'It's too painful, I just can't.' He had straightened enough for me to see that his right shoulder was not the same as the left. It was obviously dislocated. I checked the pulse on his right wrist and felt his hands. His pulse was strong and his hand warm. No circulation problems there … yet.

Not all shoulder dislocations are obvious, especially in the hospital setting where we see people of all ages and sizes. The size of a person can make it difficult to tell. Often frail people don't even need to have an accident or any overt force involved to dislocate a joint, and their statures make it hard to see if something's out of sorts. But a seventeen-year-old boy on the basketball team is likely to be tall and skinny. The poor lad didn't have enough flesh on him to hide anything.

My clinic was only 100 metres away and with the help of Brian and James we managed to get Steve lying on the examination table. I tried calling Dr Fritz but got no answer. I remembered that this was one of the few weekends he had off; we were alone.

'Fuck!' Steve was trying to find a comfortable position but not succeeding. 'Just fucking do something, fuck, fuck, fuck …' He carried on screaming, pleading, while I didn't have the courage to tell him that there was no doctor.

Steve had found the best position to ease the pain a little. He was lying face down on the examination table with his right arm hanging down off the side. 'Please do something soon. I can't take this anymore.'

In such instances the emergency call was directed to the next village over, usually a thirty-minute drive away. The next option was the ambulance, but the nearest ambulance was forty minutes away, which would mean at least an hour and a half before he got to hospital. My other option was to take him by car, screaming all the way. With such limited and unappealing choices, I opted for driving.

'Please, I can't move. Don't touch me. I can't move.' We couldn't get Steve to move off the bed let alone into a car. He'd found himself in a slightly less agonising position and was not going to budge. I needed some advice.

I try to avoid calling my colleagues, Justine and Michaela, when they're off duty because time off is supposed to be just that, and like all nurses, I know, when you ask someone for help, they will never say no. Michaela was no different and was happy to help out. In fact, Michaela relished the challenge of a decent trauma. I instantly felt reassured by her upbeat tone when she arrived.

'Don't worry about a thing,' Michaela said and quickly began examining Steve's shoulder. 'I've put dozens of shoulders back in place.' What the hell was she talking about? Nurses don't relocate limbs. At least, not nurses in Britain or New Zealand. I knew Michaela was extremely experienced and supremely confident; perhaps this is what nurses did in the States.

'What do you mean you've put in dozens of shoulders?' I whispered, thinking I was out of earshot of our patient. 'You can't do that. You're not allowed.' I know my limits, and I know what is within the scope of my practice, and what is not. Relocating the shoulder myself had never occurred to me. Steve chose that moment to scream in pain.

'Let her bloody fix it. I can't take this anymore. Just do it,' he managed to shout.

Watching someone in agony never gets any easier, and it's a whole lot worse when you don't have an IV line to insert with a whole lot of morphine or midazolam.

I was trying to think of what could go wrong if Michaela went ahead and fixed his shoulder. She could worsen any possible fracture or nerve damage, although there was no way to judge how much damage we could do by leaving him as he was – there were possible circulation problems to worry about – and this was without even considering the possibility of the relocation not working.

'We can't leave him like this for the next hour and we can't take him to the hospital. We have no choice.' Michaela was in total control, and not in the slightest bit fazed by the chaos. 'Honestly, don't worry, I've done this lots of times with the docs at work. It really does look like an uncomplicated dislocation. I know what I'm doing.'

I stood back and watched.

She rolled up a sheet, wrapped it around her waist and Steve's shoulder, and gently began to pull. 'Fuck-fuck-fuck-fuck-fuck …' Steve's screams reached new heights. I was just about to stop Michaela when … 'Thank fuck for that. Oh, thank you, thank you, thank you so much.' The relief was instant and the whole procedure over in less than ten seconds. After checking Steve's circulation and sensation in his hand, Michaela placed him in a sling and gave him some analgesia. 'I can't thank you enough,' he said repeatedly.

Part of me felt more than a little envious, the childish part that wanted to be the hero. But that was nothing to the relief I felt knowing that he was feeling so much better.

Steve was taken to the doctor the following day where an x-ray showed no fracture, and the doctor congratulated Michaela on a job well done. 'You're OK with us doing that?' I asked. I had been prepared for him to be angry with us for doing something that was a doctor's job. 'Why would I be angry? You did a good job.'

His words were not helping me to figure out what was right or wrong (if there really was any such thing), or what my exact role was. I was doing more than the average nurse, a bit of diagnosing, and administering treatments and medicines like a doctor, as well as playing detective … but nothing as practical as what Michaela had done.

Michaela's brave actions on that surprising Sunday night taught me a few lessons that I'll never forget. To act or not to act? Indeed, that is the question.

Checklist

Generally, dealing with big issues is easier, because you know it's bad, and you know you're going to need outside help. Perhaps that sounds odd, but there's no uncertainty. So much of what I see is subjective, and while kids aren't necessarily dishonest, no one is immune to playing the system.

It doesn't matter that 95 per cent of our students are either very wealthy or ridiculously wealthy, because they're all the same. They're young, impressionable, tricky, manipulative, cocky, embarrassing, awkward, fun, scared, compassionate, and clever. They're capable of anything, even fooling their favourite nurse, although I do try to catch them out when I can.

Skipping class or PE is built into their DNA, and there's no better way to achieve this goal than to pull a sickie. After my first year on the job, I'd learned, adapted, and implemented various techniques and tactics to spot the genuine from the fakes.

1. The Positive Make-Up Test.
2. Do they have a test in class? You need to be specific with your question: kids will say 'No' but get in trouble for not handing in their assignment or presentation, and when confronted

with this say, 'But you asked if I had a test, not an assignment.' I always ask the full spectrum: 'Do you have a test, assignment, homework, presentation, or anything else in class that needs to be done today, at this moment in time?'
3. *How* do they answer question 2? If they start the conversation with 'I don't have anything important in class today' I know where this is going. It sounds planned – and sick people are usually feeling too miserable to plan their escape.
4. Check with their dorm parent to see if they really were sick the night before.
5. Check the records to see if they're regularly missing a particular class, PE and Maths are particularly common.
6. Obtain as much physical data as possible. Temperature, pulse, blood pressure, bowel sounds, pallor, obvious nasal congestion, lung sounds – and document it all. By tomorrow you won't remember if they've had a cold for one day or one week, because you've seen so many students, and kids aren't the best historians, especially when they're lying.

Reading this back, it looks like I'm more of a detective than a nurse, but if that is so, then I'm the most lenient one around. It's hard to say 'no' to a desperate kid, although I can and will when required. And that's the problem with medical assessments – often the symptoms are subjective. It's much easier with injuries; give me a simple break, cut or bruise anytime.

CHAPTER TWO

Sex and Education

The talk

With children at boarding school, we end up dealing with a lot of the issues that parents usually have to deal with, and this includes relationships, hormones and sex education. We cannot ignore these issues, or hope that when the kids get home their parents give them 'the talk'. Even the most informed parents, even those still living with their children, probably have little or even no idea about the sex lives of their kids.

How on earth can parents be expected to know what's going on in their children's lives when they're thousands of miles away? I lived at home, but I still didn't have a sex talk with my dad. One day he said, 'You got hairy balls yet?' and when I turned beetroot red he handed me a book. I guess it worked for me, but I feel the kids at my school probably needed a bit more than that.

So that leaves me, your average, friendly, approachable nurse, to do the job. Am I qualified? Probably not, but I have lived. Yes, those words could certainly be taken the wrong way, but it's true. I've travelled, dated women from around the world, been a ski instructor and had women throw themselves at me (it's the uniform, not me) and even been pursued by ex-psychiatric patients. Then I got married, procreated and settled down. I also spent a few months working in a London walk-in STD clinic, so I can easily use scare tactics to terrify everyone into safe sex, even abstinence. Does this make me the best person to give our kids 'the talk'? The teachers and other faculty expect the nurses to do this, so at least they must think so, but I'll let you be the judge ...

'What feels better, sir?' asked William.

There's one in every class: someone who either knows too much, or thinks they're being clever. William was actually neither, he was simply eager.

Next to him, poor Chen had no idea what was going on. His English was good enough to learn in class, but William's question had baffled him.

I'd never meant for the friendly chat to head in this direction. I had been asked by the dorm parents in charge of the junior school to have a relaxed, almost informal discussion with the boys one evening and talk about growing up and to maybe, very gently, bring up sex. But I'd never talked to children as young as William or Chen before. They were both twelve years old and, along with the other twenty or so boys in the room, comprised all the boys who would be starting high school next year.

'It would be good to prepare them a little,' Mr Jones, the head of the junior school, had explained at the start of the year, 'so they're not completely unprepared.'

I shouldn't answer William's question. It is on my list of topics to avoid at all costs. Some of the other topics on my no-go list for talks to this age group include homosexuality, masturbation, graphic descriptions of STDs and getting in-depth and intimate about sex.

Why were these very important subjects off topic? Parents. Not all parents believe it is the school's responsibility to educate or even discuss in the most superficial manner anything regarding sex. They're concerned for the following reasons:

1. They think their child is too young to learn about sex
2. They do not think it's the job of the school to teach their children about sex
3. They worry that the teacher may unduly influence their child. A concern that is brought up nearly every time is homosexuality
4. They are worried that by talking about 'safe sex' we are encouraging their child to have sex
5. They come from places where sex is banned before marriage, and can result in imprisonment
6. Their religion does not allow it

The problem is, these kids live thousands of miles away from their parents for up to eight months a year. Some see their parents even less, as they're sent to summer school and, over Christmas, to winter camps to ski. In all the madness of such a busy life, they never get round to having 'the talk'. Even if they do, in an ideal world, it shouldn't be a 'one-off' chat, instead an ongoing dialogue – although I haven't found any teenager yet that wants such a painfully awkward thing to last longer than necessary.

These kids are curious; they sometimes have no idea what is going on with their bodies, or can't explain why they feel the way they do.

Today's talk had begun with nice safe topics – 'relationships', 'trust', ways of showing someone you liked them – but it hadn't been enough.

'What's the grossest thing you've seen?' asked Warren, our only Australian student. I gently reminded him it was not the time or place for that discussion.

'Can you get AIDS your first time?' asked João the Brazilian, his question creating quite a stir.

'Not if you use protection,' answered William.

'You get it from hookers,' said Tim, clearly a surprisingly worldly twelve-year-old.

The questions were coming thick and fast, we were way off topic, and straying into dangerous territory. But this was what they wanted to know. I had to take back control. I glanced over at their dorm parent, hoping for help, but he seemed to be enjoying the show. 'Keep going, you're doing fine,' he mouthed, although he thankfully did tell the boys to quiet down.

I decided to give them a choice. 'What do you want from me then?' I asked. 'Do you want to know about STDs, sex, or something else?'

The majority wanted to hear about STDs, although I did notice that Chen had put his hand up for all three. I asked him how much he understood, and he just wanted to know what a 'hooker' was. The lads happily volunteered this information before I had a chance to intervene.

I asked the boys to list the diseases they knew about, or had heard of. They shouted out the following:

- Warts. (William had seen one online as big as a tennis ball, and was only too happy to share the experience as well as the link to the website with us.)
- HIV. (Everyone had heard of this, but William reassured everyone that a condom would stop it.)
- Lice. (Enough of the kids had experienced head lice, and understood you could get a similar type 'down there'.)

They couldn't list any more, although they knew, for example, that there were diseases that made it painful to pee. I could have provided them with a list of diseases, but I wanted to pick up on something William had said.

'Do condoms stop disease every time?' I asked for a vote. William and a handful of others confidently put up their hand, while the rest simply didn't know.

But before I had a chance to correct them, William had asked his awkward question.

'What feels better, sir? With or without a condom?' There was silence. They leaned forward to hear my answer. Even Chen, who didn't fully understand what was being asked, sensed the question was a 'big deal' and kept quiet. Mr Jones gave me a slight nod, but this question felt too personal, so I chose to distract them.

'I was going to tell you about the kissing disease,' I began, 'but if you'd rather hear about …' I didn't finish the sentence, everyone's face had a look of horror.

'There's no kissing disease!' insisted a suddenly uncertain William.

There were some very worried faces around the room, as well as some very confused ones.

I began to talk about herpes, otherwise known as a cold sore. Nearly everyone knew about cold sores and weren't worried. But when I said that boys or girls with a cold sore could spread it 'down there' they were horrified.

I didn't help matters when I told them that condoms are not perfect. 'They reduce the chance of infection … but nothing is 100 per cent.' The poor kids were never going to kiss a girl ever, let alone have sex. It was time to ease their suffering. I began to talk about what I had planned to discuss all along: relationships, friendships, getting to know someone, learning to trust.

'If I went to a bar in town and kissed every girl in the bar, would I have a good chance of catching something?' They agreed that the chances would be high.

'Whereas if I met one girl I liked, and spent time getting to know her, came to trust her, and I kissed her, then I'd probably be OK. The most important advice I can give you is this: it all comes down to knowing someone, and eventually trusting that someone special.'

I've since learned from attending sex education courses that it was wrong of me to impose my values on the kids, but with them still being so young, it's better to instil the ideal of having one committed relationship than multiple uncommitted ones. I assumed they'd want to kiss girls, and I didn't mention same sex attraction, but I still don't know that I would bring this subject up. It's not because I think it unnecessary, but with half a dozen nationalities in the class, it's safer for the kids and for me to keep it as uncomplicated as possible … although I can't say I've ever met an uncomplicated teenager.

It's not perfect, but I feel like I'm doing some good, which is better than no good at all.

It's a bit daunting to think that I'm one of the main people of influence at this moment in the students' lives. Often no one else is telling them the things they need to know, answering their awkward questions or allaying their fears. For a lot of the children, the Christmas or spring break with their parents is too long to wait for an explanation because they're experiencing things right now. They're all growing up, some much faster than others, they're all changing, and insatiably curious.

This was not my first, and certainly not my last awkward conversation about sex with these boys. As I watched the students grow, my role expanded from school nurse to confidant and, well, you wouldn't believe some of the things I've heard! Things were about to get much stickier …

Girl talk

When it comes to sex education, I am mostly enlisted to talk to the male students, which is probably good as I have a habit of saying the wrong thing. But sometimes I don't have a choice ...

'You have to see them,' insisted Sarah, the dorm parent of the senior girls' dormitory. I turned to my colleague, Michaela.

'Does it have to be tonight?' Michaela asked. She wasn't eager to talk to the girls either, it was Friday evening and we both had the night off. Sarah was adamant that her dorm desperately needed our input, she even used the term 'emergency', but I still wasn't convinced.

I have lost count of the many 'emergencies' I have been in; some were real, some imagined, and some just plain ridiculous. I think interpretation of an emergency comes down to the various life experiences of the people involved.

My problem is that I don't like saying 'no'. In this case, I tried to come up with a semi-legitimate excuse. 'We've been drinking,' I said, indicating the half-empty bottle of red on the table. Sure, we had only had one glass each, but I was desperate for a polite way out. Still, Sarah insisted that the matter was urgent and could not wait.

'What exactly do you want us to tell them?' By asking this question I had basically admitted defeat, and Sarah sensed this too.

'Sex,' she said. 'They need a crash course in sex.'

I choked on my wine while Michaela laughed.

I've never given an 'emergency' sex talk before. Exactly what was Sarah expecting the girls to do that night? And what could I say that would make any difference? Was I supposed to discourage them from doing it? Was that even allowed? Perhaps I'm just supposed to encourage them to 'play safe'.

As a school nurse, sex education is just part of the job. It's strange how people think that just because you're a nurse, you're qualified to talk about anything physical. There is a difference between being a nurse who communicates one-to-one with a patient, and actually teaching a class. But I usually get by. I worked in an STD clinic before, so I did have some 'hands on' experience.

'Can't this wait till Monday?' Michaela asked. It could wait, but non-medical people often get worried about things that really aren't urgent, and Sarah was convinced that this was the best time; in her defence, there had been a high number of 'incidents' this year.

These included:

- A complaint from some locals living near the school about a boy getting blow jobs between morning classes, on a regular basis. The couple obviously thought the bushes behind the car park safe, but they forgot that they live on a slope, and that people living above them can see everything. The neighbours were able to give a very accurate description of the boy's face. It also explained why Johan the Swede was always late but cheerful in classes.

- A close call with a Hepatitis C epidemic. Fortunately this was a false alarm, but while we were waiting for the blood results we did have to track down all sexual contacts. The chain of connection showed that nearly every sexually active

person in the school had a sexual link to everyone else.
- A build-up of used condoms on the terrace outside the boys' dormitory.
- Three boys suspended for having spent the night in the girls' dorm.
- A hidden 'sex-pad', which was discovered in the attic of the school hall. It had been furnished with mattresses, candles, refreshments and several packets of condoms.

The frightening thing was that for every problem we knew about, there were bound to be two more we didn't, so, with a sigh, Michaela and I agreed to do the talk together.

On our way out the door Michaela grabbed some condoms and told me to bring the bananas from her kitchen.

Our strategy was simple; Michaela would talk about sex from a woman's perspective, and I'd agree with everything she said. Nothing should go wrong.

'What's he doing here?' we were asked on arrival. The voice sounded American and belonged to a blonde lass in the front row.

'Don't complain, this should be interesting,' replied her neighbour.

'Do we get to practise on him?' said another, and the room erupted in laughter.

My face turned red. What on earth was I doing? I had walked into the lion's den and I had nothing to appease these seventeen- and eighteen-year-old women. I didn't feel like an educator. If anything, I was sure I was the one about to get the education. 'I can't do this,' I whispered to Michaela. She'd be fine doing this with Sarah, without me.

'No bloody way. You're not deserting me now,' she whispered back.

I've faced some pretty hairy things during my time in the emergency room, but I've never felt as vulnerable as I did right then. The girls were giggling, chatting, even pointing. I resisted the urge to look down and make sure my fly was done up.

'Right ladies, settle down,' Sarah began. 'We've got two special guests tonight who have kindly given up their time to talk to you this evening. Please make them feel welcome.' There was a brief round of applause before we got to work.

Michaela and Sarah took two steps back, leaving me stranded.

'Right, well, so ... I hear that you need some educating about boys,' I began.

'We know all about boys,' said the American blonde in the front, her manner smug, her eyes searching the crowd for support.

'Give him a chance, Skylar,' someone from the back responded. 'I've never had a sex talk by a man before. Let's hear what men think about girls.'

I wasn't there to tell them what men think about girls, or was I? 'You want me to tell you what guys think about?' I asked. That was exactly what they wanted to know. This was an easy one to answer. But should I give the truth, or the watered-down version?

'Men are simple creatures,' I began, my mind suddenly blank. I paused and looked over at Michaela and Sarah, and they nodded at me to continue. They seemed as eager as the girls to hear what I had to say.

'Men are simple creatures,' I started again. 'They only ever think about one thing, and will tell you anything to get *it*. They'll tell lies, and they'll even tell lies honestly believing that what they are saying is the truth.'

Skylar, the blonde in the front row, interrupted. 'What do they want? What exactly is "it" you mean?' She was enjoying every minute of this.

I suddenly felt shy saying the word 'sex' in front of them. It was irrational, but I feared my voice would crack, my face turn even more beetroot, or even giggle.

'You know, they'll say anything to get you to play ...' I was about to say 'play around' but that was too ambiguous. There was a long pause as I thought of a harmless way to say sex.

'They'll say anything to get you to play hide the sausage,' I blurted.

Sarah's mouth dropped, along with everyone else's in the room, but I ploughed on.

'Perhaps that was a sexist thing to say,' I said, my tone apologetic. 'I hear women these days are just as aggressive at pursuing men.'

'He didn't just say that.' I overheard Sarah as she whispered in Michaela's ear, but it was too late now.

'Maybe I should tell the boys that you'll say anything to get what you want. Perhaps I should be warning the boys to stay away from you lot,' I said, deliberately making eye contact with Skylar. By this stage Michaela and Sarah were in an agony of laughter, along with the rest of the room. I wanted to hide, but I couldn't stop.

While many of these girls were already sexually active, they weren't adults. Just because they'd had oral sex or regular intercourse, they still had a lot to learn. Being able to physically do something has nothing to do with being mentally prepared, and especially nothing to do with being safe.

It doesn't help that the school doesn't want to deal with sex education, although that could be a good thing. When Michaela had suggested that we stock some condoms in the health centre, the headmaster had initially said 'Why? They're not having sex.' This may sound unbelievable, but sometimes it's easier to deny there is an issue, because then they don't have to deal with it.

Other than what students learn in biology class, there is no plan, no policy or goal when it comes to educating them about the birds and the bees. It's easier to leave it to the nurses, because – apparently – we know best!

'Who's had herpes before?' I asked the girls. No one was really sure. I asked if any of them had had a cold sore, and most of them raised their hand. 'Well don't kiss your boyfriend down there if you've got one, he won't forgive you. He'll have it for life.' There were gasps of disbelief. 'You're telling me you didn't know that? It works both ways, except it's usually worse for the women if they get it down there. So watch out.'

Due to the previous Hepatitis C scare, most the senior students knew about that, as well as Hepatitis A and B.

I asked them about syphilis, warts, HIV, gonorrhoea; they knew nothing, and they began to realise that they knew nothing. When I told them that we were down to the last antibiotic to treat gonorrhoea, and that pretty soon we'd have nothing to treat it, they were ready to listen. Even Skylar managed to keep her mouth shut.

I told them about my experiences working at a London STD clinic. The biggest lesson I learned from that place was not to judge anyone by appearances. In the waiting room you'd see the most sophisticated, beautifully dressed men and women, sitting next to someone more used to sleeping on the street, and they usually had something in common – an STD.

I was surprised when one young teen said that we didn't need to worry about STDs so much in our village, because we lived in the Alps. She seemed to think that our location was some protection from STDs. I soon explained how wrong she was; ski resorts have a disproportionate number of STD cases. 'And besides, I see cases from school every year with STDs.' There were horrified gasps alongside demands to know who they were.

Another girl thought that oral and anal sex were safe alternatives to regular sex.

'Hands up if you think you can catch a disease from oral sex.' Only half the girls raised their hands.

'A friend told me ...' began another. It's always a friend, or a friend of a friend, but it doesn't matter. I listened. This particular friend thought that anal sex meant the person was still a virgin. I'd never thought about it before, but I guess technically you could say that. 'But bugs can spread particularly easily through anal sex,' I explained. 'It's why we often give people their medicine that way.'

With my credentials established, the girls wanted to know more. They asked a whole range of questions:

- How do you know when it's right?
- My friend has a boyfriend who is going to dump her if she doesn't 'do it'. Should she?
- Do condoms always stop disease?
- Can you cure genital warts?
- Can you get cancer?
- Is it always painful?
- What's a normal size? (Penis size, that is.)
- Is anal sex safe?
- What is dogging?
- What is chariot racing? (I had to look this up on Google, although I advise you not to.)

Their appetite was insatiable, but finally we were finished, and we let the girls go, free to pursue or be pursued. Sarah came over and thanked us. She said that in her time as a dorm parent she'd never seen such an 'enthusiastic' response to a sex talk. I just hoped that I still had a job come Monday morning.

When Monday finally came around, instead of angry phone calls or vicious emails, I was approached by a group of senior boys. They asked when their sex talk was. They said they'd heard from the girls that it was the best sex education talk ever. I think they felt left out of all the fun.

As politically incorrect and potentially offensive as my tactics may sound, over the years that I've been a school nurse, I've discovered humour nearly always helps.

A lot of students come to me now, especially after I give a group lesson, to speak privately. It's during these talks that I realise how little they truly know and how important it is that we continue to communicate.

Teaching the teachers

We needed some guidance. After my first two sexual education talks, I had many unanswered questions:

- What is appropriate for a ten-year-old versus someone sixteen years or older?
- Should we even be offering sex education to everyone?
- Do we talk about homosexuality? And how do we handle such a sensitive subject given the backgrounds of some of our kids?
- Do we need parental consent?
- Could we get into trouble?
- What should you expect ten-to sixteen-year-olds to know? Is there a baseline of understanding, a bare minimum they should know?
- And how much is an average teenager exposed to, compared to when I was at school? Do they learn it all on the internet?

To help us in our quest to provide relevant, age appropriate, unbiased information, we went on a research trip to London. Britain has had boarding schools for hundreds of years, and, I like to think, pretty much have them sorted. These institutions have heaps of resources for matrons, nurses, dorm parents and teachers. Our brief was three-fold. Michaela, Justine and I went to a conference all about sexual education; we invited a sexual education specialist to come to our school and educate us about how to teach; and we invested in pamphlets, booklets, questionnaires, DVDs and online resources to make our lessons more interesting and, as far as possible, more 'hands on'.

With all this new material, I now felt better prepared, but it wasn't until my second year that I got to do another sex talk, and it happened to include some of the boys from my first: William, Chen and João. They had made the transition from junior school to high school, and the powers that be felt it a good idea to follow up from the previous year's talk. They set aside the boys' common room one evening for me to do my thing.

This time I was armed to the hilt. I had a questionnaire, a five-minute video on dating and even props.

'What's in the box, sir?' William asked, as eager as ever. I wanted to keep the props for the 'hands-on' part at the end, but the boys were too distracted for my quiz, so I popped the lid and delved inside.

'Contraception is all about correct technique,' I said, handing the first penis to William.

'No way, that's disgusting,' cried João.

'It's a bit small, sir,' William observed.

'Nah, that size seems about right for you,' said another boy.

According to the guidelines, we're supposed to teach proper technique, and make sure the boys know how to put a condom on, take one off and dispose of it.

I reached down to pick up another prop.

'Get it out of my face, you homo,' shouted João as William tried to insert his prop into his friend's mouth.

'You seem to be enjoying playing with that, Will,' I observed, before admonishing him for his choice of language, and he quickly cut out his antics.

I handed the next penis to João.

It would have been better if they'd sent us penises all the same size. João's was a good two inches bigger than William's.

'Now you're talking,' he crowed. All twelve boys doubled up with laughter.

I'd started so well, and now it was a circus.

'What about me, sir? You got one big enough for me?' said Nnakeme. I knew this would happen – boys will be boys – but I was committed now and ploughed ahead.

'Who knows how to put on a condom?'

João volunteered, and he didn't do too badly.

After showing them how to put a condom on and remove it properly, they all had a go, no one was exempt, whatever their background.

It was a fun way to start the session, but now it was time for something a bit more serious, and I handed them the test I'd borrowed from the conference I'd been to in England. They said it was 'age appropriate' for 3rd form boys and approved for use in British schools. I was doing everything by the book. Nothing could go wrong.

The Test

The boys needed to answer 'True', 'False' or 'Unsure' to the following statements:

1. A woman can't get pregnant the first time she has sex
2. A woman can't get pregnant if the man pulls out before he ejaculates
3. When a girl says no, she doesn't always mean it

4. You can tell if someone has a sexually transmitted disease
5. Only gay men are at risk of HIV
6. If you love someone you shouldn't have to use a condom
7. Girls can't get contraception until they are sixteen years old
8. If a girl is on the pill it means she's easy
9. Two men or women can be in love with each other
10. It is better to wait until marriage before having sex
11. Someone has to sleep around to get an STD
12. Someone can get an STD from oral sex
13. Using a condom can protect against HIV and STDs

I struggle to think what I would have answered when I was thirteen. We certainly had nothing like this test when I was a boy. But the results of this test, and the many times I've conducted it since, make me think that perhaps students do need such information at such a tender and impressionable age.

1. Three boys said you can't get pregnant the first time, and in every group I've since asked, there's always one or two that get this wrong.

2. A woman can get pregnant if the man pulls out. On average half the class get this wrong.

3. No means 'No'. Worryingly, on average 3–4 out of twelve get this wrong. I use this opportunity to talk about rape, statutory rape, and problems with consent when alcohol is involved, and knowing the laws of the country you are in.

4. You can't always tell if someone has an STD. Nearly everyone gets this right.

5. One or two will say 'true' and a few will say 'maybe'. They really do think HIV is a 'gay only' disease.

6. The majority get this right and say 'false'.

7. Most get this wrong, and don't realise someone under sixteen years of age can be on some form of contraception.

8. Being on the pill doesn't mean she's 'easy'. In one class, half the kids answered 'true' or 'maybe'. I also explained that not all people who take oral contraceptives take it for that purpose.

9. There are always, at least, two or three who say two men or two women cannot love each other.

10. Even those from stern religious backgrounds often feel that you shouldn't wait until marriage before having sex. I do say there is no right or wrong answer for this.

11. There are always some 'maybes' and the occasional 'true', but they were shocked to discover that people can have HIV and have never slept around.

12. A lot of kids think oral sex is safe; often over half the class answer 'false' or 'maybe'.

13. While condoms do protect against HIV and STDs, a lot of it comes down to good technique. None of the kids knew that nothing is 100 per cent.

I had some very interesting results. The information gave me some idea of what they needed to know, and in some cases, showed me how they might need to change their attitude. Of course it's not for me to unduly influence, but boys who genuinely believe a girl doesn't always mean 'no' when she says it, could end up in a lot of trouble one day.

Kurt and Rachel

Rachel burst into my office, gasping for air. She had run all the way from the school theatre to get here. It's not far, but it's uphill.

'Sir, you have to come quick, please, it's urgent.'

I asked what was wrong, but Rachel just grabbed my hand and began pulling me out of the office. 'Please, sir, just come quick … Kurt is hurt real bad, there's blood everywhere.' I let her lead me out of the office, making sure to bring my emergency bag.

As Rachel lead me through the theatre, past the empty stalls, and behind the stage, I wondered where the hell I was going to end up, and what they'd been doing. I'd never been backstage before, but Rachel knew exactly where she was going. She lead into the boys' changing room.

Kurt was in a bad state. He was lying on the floor, next to the sink. His pants were down around his ankles, and there was blood on his head as well as on the floor, although I couldn't tell exactly where all the blood was coming from. There seemed to be more than one source of bleeding. Fortunately Kurt was conscious, although as pale as a sheet.

'What's wrong, mate, what happened?' I asked as I knelt down beside him. He lay still but turned his eyes towards me.

'I feel shit,' he croaked as he tried to sit up, but I told him to stay lying until I'd had a chance to examine him.

He tried to pull up his pants and I helped him cover himself, while Rachel looked away, her face reddening. 'I was standing up, then woke up on the floor,' he said. I asked what he was doing at the time, and he glanced at Rachel and gave her an almost imperceptible nod.

'We were …' Rachel stuttered, 'we were doing, you know … it. And then he screamed, and there was blood, down there. His … his dick was bleeding.' Kurt was feeling a bit better and again tried to move to a sitting position. I told him to lie back down as I needed to make sure his head and neck were fine but he sat up anyway. 'It's so fucking sore.' I assumed he meant his head, but he very slowly put his hands in his pants and gently cradled his penis.

'Mate, what have you done?' I managed a quick glance and it looked a mess.

'She broke it.'

Rachel began sobbing.

'I'm sorry, I never meant to, I'm sorry.'

'Is it gonna be OK, Doc?' asked Kurt.

I imagined saying 'No' to make sure Kurt got the most out of the experience, but my usual kidding around didn't seem the best course of action. There was a lot of blood down there and while I couldn't make out what exactly was wrong, I felt sure it wouldn't be serious – simply because I didn't have the imagination to come up with something overly worrying that could have happened.

In hindsight he could have had a fractured penis, something I'd only read about being possible, and had no idea what such a thing would look like! With all the blood I felt certain Kurt's problem was probably more superficial.

Kurt denied any neck or back pain, although he did have a three-centimetre laceration above his right eyebrow. I wrapped a bandage around his head and walked him slowly back to the health centre whereupon I received the whole story.

'We didn't warm up, it's my fault,' Rachel began while Kurt lay back on the couch, still cradling his manhood as he moaned in agreement.

'Yeah, it's her fault.'

They'd snuck off to the theatre changing rooms for a quickie between classes. 'The floor was so gross,' Rachel said, 'so we did it standing up.'

'She split my dick in half,' Kurt cut in. I hoped that wasn't the case. It was time to take a proper look at it, so I gloved up and shooed Rachel out the room.

'Softly, Doc. Softly.' Kurt gently lowered his pants and tenderly laid out his willy. The poor thing looked like it had been through a war, blood and all, but I could see the problem. I breathed a sigh of relief.

'It's OK, you've only split your foreskin in half.'

'What do you mean *only split it in half*,' Kurt exclaimed, his voice cracking, close to tears. Perhaps I shouldn't have said 'you've only', as I've never had such an injury, especially considering the pain had been so bad that he had a vasovagal episode, which caused the faint, whereupon he hit his head against the sink on the way to the floor.

Most fainting by young healthy people is vasovagal. The vagal nerve runs from the head through the middle of the body. When this nerve is stimulated, as it was by the pain from his split foreskin, it slows the pulse down – a lot – from 80 beats per minute to zero beats per minute. Only briefly, of course, otherwise you'd be dead. But the subsequent drop in pressure allows gravity to take effect, and your blood pressure ends up in your boots. The good news is that when you hit the ground, you end up in a lying position, which helps the blood pressure return to normal. There are many things that stimulate this nerve, and pain is a very common one.

Poor Rachel had received such a fright at the suddenness of Kurt's collapse that she thought she had 'shagged him to death'.

Kurt's mood slowly improved, although he still spent the next two hours cradling his penis. He was nauseous, pale, and would need four stitches to his forehead.

We eventually had him reviewed by the village doctor. His bleeding parts were patched up and he was kept in the health centre for the night for observation.

While Kurt may not want to speak of his experience for a few years ... I'm sure when he's older both he and Rachel will relish retelling the story of how he was almost shagged to death. Men enjoy these stories of past and mighty conquests. And of course, as the saying goes, if you're going to die, you might as well go out with a bang ...

Night-time wanderings

It's not just the kids that have a hard time finding privacy. Young, free and single faculty members have to be careful as well. Sean's story was a lesson to us all.

The witching hour is usually considered midnight, but it's more like 5.30am at boarding school. This is when all manner of creatures emerge from their dens of sin and scuttle home to hide their shame just before sunrise. It's the time that Sean deemed it safe enough to risk an escape and make a run for it.

It never looks good for a male teacher to be seen leaving the female dorm area in the middle of the night. But what else could he do? He'd met the woman of his dreams, Sasha, a pretty maths teacher. He wouldn't have been in trouble if his budding relationship had been public knowledge, or even for staying the night, they were both adults. Sometimes I think it's simply because there are no secrets in boarding school that people try to keep them.

Marco also thought 5.30am was a safe time to escape the girls' dorm, taking the above-ground path to safety, walking somewhat dangerously across the rooftops.

Stephanie chose the same route but was leaving the boys' dorm, coming across the roof from the east, while the two males were coming from the west.

Their paths inevitably crossed: one teacher, two students.

There would be repercussions for everyone.

Marco was suspended for two weeks, Stephanie for one. Sean was more fortunate; in fact, it got their relationship out in the open and, many years later, he ended up marrying Sasha.

Marco's punishment was more severe because he'd stolen a dorm key to enter the building, while Stephanie had been smuggled into the boys' dorm in her boyfriend's suitcase. The staff had even helped enable this feat by letting the boyfriend use the elevator. If only kids used these smarts in the classroom!

Sean did admit that he was very briefly tempted to pretend he'd never seen the others on the roof that night, especially when Marco offered him a deal: 'You don't see me, and I don't see you,' but he made the right choice.

It wasn't all bad for Marco and Stephanie. Few escapades gain such instant fame amongst peers as rooftop wanderings in the dead of night.

The sex side of things

For both the staff and the students, it's hard to have a private life at a boarding school – you really have to make an effort to be alone.

For staff, being 'off duty' doesn't mean a thing to the kids when you live in the same building, the same floor, the same corridor. Whether it's a harmless secret, or something more *interesting*, you'll eventually get found out.

For the students, finding a place to have some one-on-one time is never easy. I have to hand it to the older kids, they are certainly creative in finding solutions:

- Renting a local apartment for the *year* to use as a party, sex, smoking and drinking pad.
- Building a forest hut, able to withstand the rain, but not the snow; great for the summer months.
- Visiting the local cave – a thirty-minute hike, but that's nothing for two lusting teenagers!

How do I find these things out? I don't go looking, and I really don't want to know, but I don't always have a choice.

The crush

It's nice to feel appreciated; it only takes a kind word or gesture to transform an average day, or even an awful day, into a bright one. Something as simple as a kind note left on your desk can work wonders. But things can often turn complicated when dealing with adolescents.

Chocolates are a relatively simple gift (as long as they're not Russian, they taste awful). Chocolates are my go to present when I want to make a gesture of appreciation.

Alcohol is a common gift to staff from students – each nationality brings me their country's best. From any student from Eastern Europe, vodka is the weapon of choice, with every vodka-producing nation naturally insisting its product is the best. From the Mexican students, it's always tequila; cachaça from the Brazilians; and single malt whisky for most of the Western nations, as well as, perhaps surprisingly, the Saudi students.

Usually parents buy the gift and send their child to school loaded with hard spirits. The gesture is always appreciated, and the child is proud to show off the finest alcohol their nation can produce.

But sometimes people want to give more.

Teenagers are spontaneous, their emotions high one moment, low the next. Their feelings are intense and these little gifts of appreciation are sometimes just not a big enough gesture.

How can they find a way to express their gratitude to the person who changed their failing grade from a D to a B, especially when school is not just the biggest thing in their life at that time, it *is* their whole life? How can they thank the person who comforted them when they were homesick, or helped them fit in and make friends?

'I can't thank you enough. You're the best' – the note was signed 'Priscilla'. The letter was for my friend, Brian, a maths teacher.

'She worked for it,' Brian said. 'She went to every extra help session I gave, and still wanted more.' Brian explained that she had been willing to pay for private lessons on top of the regular after school group sessions, but he'd refused. 'You turned down 100 euros an hour?' Maths and physics teachers were always in demand, and tutors could get away with charging such a heavy fee.

'That's actually why I'm here,' Brian said. 'I wanted your expert opinion.' I motioned for him to continue. 'Is she ADHD or something?' he asked. 'Or seeing the counsellor for any issues?' I asked him why he thought she might have 'issues' and to tell me exactly what she does that makes him think so.

Many teachers have concerns about their students, and often say things like 'she's ADHD' or describe someone as 'bipolar'. Even the most well-meaning people throw these terms out there, and nearly every time it's wrong, but labels can stick. I need to find out what the student is actually doing that is causing concern.

Do they talk non-stop in class? Do they interrupt others? Are they aggressive or act like a bully? Do they do their work? Do they say strange things?

Priscilla, Brian explained, did all of the above, particularly constantly talk in class, disturb others, and struggle with work – hence the extra help to enable her to pass Maths. Like many fifteen-year-old girls, she lived her life as if on a permanent emotional rollercoaster. Fortunately for her, and us, it was a rollercoaster with peaks of pure joy, and not particularly deep lows.

But it wasn't this behaviour that bothered him, as it's pretty normal. 'She follows me ... *everywhere,*' he added. Priscilla had changed her activity from volleyball (which she loved) to hiking (which Brian led). 'She won't stop staring at me in class, and is always the last to leave. She's even got her mum on her side, insisting I continue with her private lessons. She's obsessed. She's even said she's got a surprise for my birthday next week.'

I promised to pass on his concerns to the counsellor, although I didn't think the matter urgent. 'A bit of a crush,' I remember saying so clearly. No one could have anticipated the surprise she had in store for him.

It wasn't just any birthday, it was Brian's fortieth and understandably his students enjoyed teasing him about becoming officially old (or 'ancient', as they called it). Priscilla didn't join in the banter, instead she enlisted the help of her peers.

As Brian turned up to class the following week on the day of his birthday, he did what he always did at the start of a lesson and took the register. Everyone was present bar one. When he called out 'Priscilla' the music began.

Priscilla entered the room, dressed in a flimsy white dress, and began to sing happy birthday. It wasn't your typical 'happy birthday' where everyone joins in. Priscilla must have seen Marilyn Monroe singing happy birthday to a naughty president at some stage, and thought Brian would appreciate the gesture.

What does one do when confronted by a flirtatious teenager?

You politely interrupt, say 'thank you' and explain that the classroom is not the right place for such behaviour.

Of course, it's not always that easy. 'She was so serious,' Brian described later, 'it would've crushed her if I'd made her stop straight away.' Instead, he ended up saying things like 'it's unique' and 'unforgettable' while trying to avoid actual words of encouragement.

Priscilla cut her performance short, but she was not discouraged, and after being sent away to get changed, she came back ready for the grand finale.

It was the last class of the day, and Priscilla waited until everyone had left the room, whereupon she threw herself at Brian.

Brian disentangled himself from her clutches and sprinted to the headmaster's office.

Priscilla did see the counsellor, that same day. She was immediately transferred to another Maths class, and her mother notified.

Fortunately, Priscilla wasn't too upset, or overly embarrassed, which is unusual, and she quickly stopped pursuing Brian. Her new maths teacher, Mr Cooper, seemed a bit nervous when she asked him for extra lessons but by that time I think Priscilla had grown out of teenage infatuation and started dating someone her own age. Ah, teenage love – how quickly it can come … and go!

Using your assets

Some kids will go to any lengths to get what they want.

'Sir, can I ...' Stacey asked.

'No.'

'But you haven't ...'

'No.'

It's very educational watching a teenager's reaction when you not only give them an answer they don't want to hear, but don't give them a chance to finish. This may sound cruel, but Stacey was supposed to be in class. She was physically well, and she knew better. She had been at the school for three years, yet even at nearly nineteen years of age, she still stretched the rules. I explained to her that as it wasn't urgent, she could come and see me during the designated clinic times. Seeing how a person reacts tells me a lot about who they are and what they've learned from their parents.

The reactions come in a variety of forms, most of them unpleasant. Sometimes the pupil storms out, slamming the door; others beg and plead; some just refuse to leave; a portion of them will dial their parents and hand their phone to me (I no longer accept phone calls from parents in this particular situation); a rare few simply accept that they should be in class, and quietly leave without putting up a fight.

I know teenagers are difficult, and I do worry about my own children when they get to that age. I worry that I'm tempting fate by judging too harshly, but I have standards. I was a good teenager. I never spoke back and I never slammed doors. I did what was asked, and if I disagreed with a teacher, I'd talk about it with my parents later that evening. If my parents agreed, they'd contact the school and discuss the matter rationally, without shouting or threats. This 'normal' behaviour is becoming rare, not just in elite boarding schools, but in your average public school.

What only a handful of the students at my school realise is that if they're nice, I give in. I let them have their Strepsils, lip balm, or moisturiser, before heading back to class. These are not exactly urgent needs, and the student should be made to wait until the appropriate time, but I can't say no when they're polite enough.

Stacey was a challenge for me because she was polite and insistently apologetic.

'Please … I'm sorry … you have to help.' What was I doing so wrong that children had to plead with me? 'It won't take long, but it's urgent.' She looked ready to cry.

Within a few months of working as a school nurse, I realised I have a talent for making girls burst into tears. Ten years later I've become used to it, but I'm still not immune. Besides, how can I refuse someone with an 'urgent' health problem? I had to at least find out what was going on with Stacey, even though she looked well and healthy. Apologising some more, she made it into my office and sat down opposite me.

Historically, whenever Stacey had made it this far into the health centre, she always got what she wanted. She knew she already had me.

She started: 'I can't go skiing this afternoon …' I cut her off, 'You said it was urgent.'

Any sign of those 'tears' that had seemed so close before had disappeared. 'How do you expect me to ski when I've hurt my bad knee?'

All kids have a bad something, whether it's a knee, ankle, or back, which always seem to flare up when the clouds roll in and the temperature drops; they're like old grandmas.

The problem with knees is that they usually look fine, so it becomes a matter of trust, of which I had none when it came to Stacey.

I reminded her again that we were only to see urgent problems outside clinic times, but she chose not to understand. 'Please, it is urgent. You have to excuse me.'

Stacey leaned forward as she pleaded with me, and I was willing to give her a break, just to get her out of my office. Here we hit the crux of the matter.

To Stacey, as well as most teenage girls, school uniforms are not something to take pride in, but something to be manipulated into showing as much of their body as possible. Stacey, for example, had more than the normal number of buttons on her blouse undone, and I found myself staring out the window, at the ceiling, anywhere that was not in her direction because when she leaned forward, on the already low chair, with half her buttons undone, well … you can understand my discomfort. This was not a new tactic and most of her male teachers had said it's easier just to give her what she wants and get her out the room as quickly as possible.

That was Stacey's *modus operandi*. She would plead politely, then expose, plead again and expose again. I didn't know where to look. I never did. I was tired of feeling uncomfortable whenever she came into my office.

To make matters even worse, Stacey would also hike her skirt up even higher than most of the girls. Normally it's rolled up four inches or so around the hips.

I couldn't go on working like this. At eighteen years of age, Stacey was fully developed and with her make-up on looked like someone in their mid-twenties. If you saw her at a pub, anyone would mistake her for a mature adult.

I was being manipulated, and we both knew she had the upper hand. But I was sick of her behaviour. I decided to take control. This stopped now.

'Stacey, do you not know how to dress?' She sat back in her chair, feigning shock, her hands folded on her lap.

'What do you mean?'

I had no choice, but to be blunt. 'Stacey, you need to do the buttons up on your top.'

She didn't move. 'I know how to dress fine. It's not my fault you're uncomfortable.' She actually looked down at her chest when she said this.

'I can see nearly everything, and when you lean forward I can see the rest. You need to do up your top, now.' She still didn't make a move to do up her top buttons, instead she leaned forward again, while looking down as if to judge just how much she did expose.

'Stacey, I'm trying to help you here. I'm a nurse. Do you know what that means?'

She shrugged her shoulders, my words having no impact.

'It means I've seen hundreds of breasts. Put them away and save them for someone else.'

'You ... you can't say that!' Stacey repeated those words as she hurriedly did up her blouse and left my office.

I never did get to look at her knee but it turned out to be nothing and she ended up having to go skiing. I never heard another peep out of her.

Stacey was not the first – or the last – young woman to try and use their feminine assets to get their way. It would also be wrong to deny that this is something I rarely have to deal with, because as a male nurse it's something I do need to be aware of, as well as be extra sensitive to the fact that I'm a male in a predominantly female profession.

I don't always know the best way to deal with some of the rules in these situations, especially the first time I encounter them, but as a general rule of thumb, I try to confront the issue as it happens – even if the only thing you want to do is run as far away as possible.

Long weekends

'My flight is booked, I have to go. Please,' Mary pleaded. Mary had booked a flight to Barcelona for a long weekend to celebrate her sixteenth birthday. 'I'm going to be with my parents the whole time. I won't be doing anything bad.'

Mary had recently been caught lying to us. She had come to my office and claimed she was sick and couldn't play sport, but later that evening had been caught leaving one of the local restaurants, cigarette in hand. The punishment for her deception was that she was not allowed to travel for the long weekend and had to serve detention.

But things are never simple in boarding schools. With the airfare already booked, and the parents arguing that the school was being unfair, the headmaster had left the decision up to me – the original victim of Mary's lies – to decide if she could travel on the long weekend, and have her punishment deferred to the following weekend.

'This isn't the first time you've been caught lying to us, Mary,' I said, raising my eyebrow to silence her when she started to protest. 'I think this is a lesson you need to learn. You can't keep abusing the health centre.'

Mary changed tack.

'I know I've not been good. But I've really learned my lesson. Please, sir, please let me go.' As I mentioned earlier, I'm a sucker for polite pleading. I really did want to let her go. I had hoped the headmaster would not leave the decision to me. I'm a nurse, not a headmaster, and I'm often a pushover. Mary sensed my doubt and pushed her case.

'I'll do anything, sir, anything you want.' I told her to stop there. I needed some time to think. But Mary wasn't finished. 'Sir, when I say anything, I mean it. I'll do *anything*.' Mary chose that moment to put her hands on her knees …

Was I imagining things, or did she pull her legs slightly apart? Was I reading more into the situation than was really there?

I panicked and chose the easiest way out. I let her go on her trip and made her promise not to come to my office again. She squealed with delight, jumped to her feet and tried hugging me, but I pulled away.

'Thank you so much, I'll never forget this,' she said, as she skipped out of the room, while I walked quickly to the headmaster's office.

'I just don't know,' I found myself saying over and over after explaining what had just happened, pacing up and down within Mr Driscoll's office. 'Was I imagining things?' There is no way to know for sure, but I've learned to trust my instincts. Being open and honest with the headmaster seemed the best course of action.

Mr Driscoll reassured me that I was not the first person to express concerns about Mary's behaviour, that a number of staff, both male and female, had mentioned her name. Often it was the little things she did that, on their own, don't seem to be too big of a deal, like being late to class once too often, or claiming illness when a test was due, or always being on the periphery of any mischief. But when all these loose ends come together, they paint quite a worrying picture. This made me feel like I made the best decision to bring it to his attention. When it comes to working alongside school kids, the best policy is always honesty … no matter how vulnerable it can make you feel.

Veronika

At eighteen years of age, Veronika was another boarding school veteran who knew how to get her way, no matter what.

'You have to see me, it's urgent,' she insisted.

It was her third visit to the health centre this week. Every time she had said it was urgent, and every time it had turned out to be nothing. The problem I have is that when people say it's urgent, I have to see them, because the one time I don't make the effort to even listen, and shoo them away, I know it really will be an emergency.

Her first urgent visit had been on Monday morning. She was worried about her shoulder. 'It's painful when I go like this.' She then swung her arm around rapidly, indicating a pain deep inside her shoulder. 'Don't swing your arm like that,' I advised her, and sent her on her way. She seemed mildly unhappy.

The second 'urgent' visit had been on Tuesday. She thought she had pneumonia because when she had woken up in the morning she had coughed up a lump of nasty looking sputum. Other than a slightly sniffly nose, she was fine, and after giving her a complete check-up (nothing less would have satisfied) she left the clinic with some nose spray. She seemed even less happy than she did the previous day.

She managed Wednesday without coming to see me, but Thursday morning she returned with a new problem.

'I need something, anything,' she pleaded. 'I haven't slept for a week.' I get a regular stream of students with sleep problems, and it's usually simple to treat:

- No sugary drinks after 5pm
- No caffeine after lunch
- No laptop, iPad, or other electronic gadget for two hours before bedtime
- One hot shower, followed by herbal tea one hour before bedtime
- A book, not a game or surfing the net, but an actual book to read for pleasure
- No study one hour before bedtime. If you haven't learned what you need for the next morning's exam, you're not going to learn it by staying up all night. You're better off getting the rest

I went through the usual steps, but Veronika refused to leave. 'You're not ignoring me this time. I want something to make me sleep.' I was about to explain that I never give sleeping pills to students, but she cut me off.

'Do you not like me?'

I reassured her I did like her but she was too worked up to listen. 'You don't give me any real medicine. Is it because I'm Russian? I know what you all think of us.'

It would be very interesting to find out what she thought we *all* thought of her. I didn't think I had anything against Russian people. I don't consider myself racist at all.

Instead of racism, I often see ignorance or simple inexperience: people who just don't know. They don't know about you, your country or your culture, resulting in some simple but painful misconceptions. Before working at an international school, I was very much one of those people who had a lot to learn about other cultures.

I had assumed that everything and everyone from Poland eastward was the same. They all drank vodka, spoke Russian (or at least sounded like they did) and had corrupt governments, often run by the mafia. My wife has only just forgiven, but never forgotten, my offhand remark during one of our rare arguments when I'd said she might as well immigrate to Moscow. My wife is Polish; I will never make that mistake again. She has also rectified many of my other misconceptions.

I had an idea.

'You're right,' I said, replying to Veronika's question. She blinked several times, slack-jawed, until it finally registered what I'd just said.

'You don't like Russians?' she asked, awed.

'I do like Russian people. I just don't know many of them.' I paused briefly, before carrying on. 'You'd like my wife. She doesn't think I'm racist, just stupid.' This brought a smile to Veronika's face. She asked if my wife was Russian.

'Polish,' I said, 'but you're all the same ... right?' Veronika was smiling now.

'Can I let you in on a secret?' I asked.

Veronika's attitude had completely changed. Here was someone not just listening, but sharing a bit of their personal life – a bit of themselves – with her. 'My wife and I always argue about how to treat our kids when they're sick. She thinks I'm crazy.'

Veronika was dying to know the details. So I told her:

My wife believes the cold will make you sick, and rarely lets the kids go barefoot about the house unless it's the height of summer. But so long as there's nothing around for them to step on, bare feet are fine by me. I said that she also believes leaving the window open at night in the winter will also make you sick. So, I secretly open the window in the middle of the night, and she secretly gets up and closes it once I've gone back to sleep. I told that I believe when treating cuts and scrapes, they're better left to the open air to dry out and heal quicker and that my wife disagrees. And, finally, that I never use 'anti-bacterial' creams on wounds. But my wife does.

For every opinion on medical care I shared about my wife, Veronika nodded in agreement.

'I'm not ignoring your problems,' I said. 'We just come from places that do things a bit differently.'

Veronika left my office and promised to try my techniques to help her get to sleep, even though I was convinced she didn't need them.

Veronika's story should end here. But, as it so often does, things then got … complicated.

Veronika stopped by on Friday to say that she had followed my advice, but had still had trouble getting to sleep the previous night. She agreed to keep at it over the weekend. I promised that I'd have some more options for her on Monday.

No one was surprised by the sight of Veronika sitting in the waiting room on Monday morning. She didn't look like someone who hadn't slept. She was cheerful, playful, and vibrant. She'd also made the effort, her make-up was immaculate.

'Did it help?' I enquired. She said my techniques helped a lot, but she wanted something more. 'Just in case I have a bad night.'

I didn't have anything concrete, no herbal teas or even medication, but what I did have was a simple self-hypnosis technique that a hypnotist, one who usually performs on stage, demonstrated to me. But, the more I thought about this option, the more I was reluctant to share it.

'I can't really show you,' I confessed, 'it wouldn't be appropriate.'

It's a simple technique, which I've used on a dozen or so of my friends, and they swear it works wonders. But when you're responsible for children, it's better to avoid techniques or tricks that I'm not professionally trained to do.

Veronika's curiosity was piqued. 'Don't you like me?' she said it teasingly this time. 'Don't you like Russians?' I shooed her out my office.

The rest of the day was uneventful, and I prepared myself for the night shift. Working the night shift meant sleeping in the health centre, with the emergency phone beside me.

At 10pm the emergency phone rang. It was the head of the girls' dorm.

'Veronika says she has to come see you tonight,' said Sarah, the dorm parent – the same dorm parent who'd insisted on an emergency sex talk. 'She said it's absolutely urgent.' Was this another 'urgent' non-issue?

I felt like Sarah was testing me. She was an experienced dorm head, and should know better than to call the emergency number for such a problem as this. 'Send her to bed. It can wait till the morning,' I said, then added: 'What do you think?'

Sarah agreed wholeheartedly, and apologised for calling so late for something so trivial.

Ten minutes later the phone rang again.

'Sir …' it was Veronika on the emergency line. 'Are you sure you don't want me to come?' Her tone was playful.

I warned her that if she used the emergency phone again, she'd get detention.

'Your loss,' she didn't sound exactly worried by my threat. She then promptly hung up.

Maybe these situations shock you, make you cringe, laugh or feel angry, but they terrify me. Working as a male nurse in the environment I do makes me vulnerable. In this particular case, I think the moment I shared a little of my personal life, about my wife and the disagreements we sometimes have, was the moment when Veronika saw me as human, and someone who cared. It's probably also when her emotions got a bit mixed, the boundaries blurred, and where she might have seen me as something more than one of the faculty members. With so many new and exciting emotions flying around inside a teenager's head, they can be forgiven for some odd flights of fancy and bad decisions, but even to this day, these moments continue to terrify me and keep me on my toes. And I think that's a good thing.

Consent

Perhaps I shared a bit much of my personal life with Veronika, but it's a strategy my nursing tutors even recommended. 'Sharing a bit of yourself helps develop rapport and trust' they said. You'd think after my experiences I would have learnt to keep my mouth shut and stay out of other people's business. But no! I still find myself poking my nose in where I shouldn't, as was the case with Corinne and Naomi. I'm convinced I was doing it for the right reasons. What do you think?

Corinne and Naomi shared everything, from their wardrobe, make-up and impetigo to their first hangover. Nothing could separate them, not even Luke, Naomi's first boyfriend. 'Chicks before dicks' they'd say before giggling like children. But they weren't really children, they were that complicated blend of wannabe adult and naïve adolescent … and blind to the dangers that come with that territory.

What fifteen-year-old child really has any understanding of the risks they take when all they're doing is having a little fun, with good people, with their friends? What harm could come from going to the city for the weekend to party with their school mates?

Everyone – staff included – knew about the upcoming Paris party; word always gets out. The staff know the students are going to get drunk, get laid, and maybe take substances they shouldn't, but their parents keep on sending their written consent for their child to go.

'They'll be with their father' or 'uncle' or 'big brother' they usually say. Sometimes this is true, sometimes not. So what can I do? They're no longer my or the school's responsibility: they've been signed out for the whole weekend. The school no longer has authority or power to stop them and we would be overstepping our bounds if we tried.

But that doesn't mean I don't still care, because every year, without fail, I get 'the call'.

'The call' is usually from a local hospital, and their patient is one of our students. There are no parents or other relatives to be found anywhere, and their only recourse is to call the school nurse. It's then that I have to make my own 'call' to the parents (if we can get hold of them).

It never gets easier telling a parent their child is in hospital or on a ventilator, or that the amount of alcohol in their child's bloodstream is enough to kill a bear, let alone a human. It's why I usually wait until I'm at the bedside and have some idea of how bad the situation is.

If it looks like the student is going to be fine, the first words out of my mouth are usually 'they're in hospital, but they're going to be OK'. Maybe I should draw out the conversation, let the dread build up – punish the irresponsible parents who happily signed their own flesh and blood over to the devil. But I don't. I'm human, and I'm a parent.

Naomi and Corinne were both going to the city to party with the boys.

Twenty boys and two girls were on the trip which meant that probably, but by no means definitely, at least eighteen boys were going to be disappointed, although not Luke. He had been mouthing off to the lads that this was the weekend him and Naomi were going to 'do it'. How did I know this? I knew because Luke couldn't keep his mouth shut. He'd told his best friend, who'd told another friend, who'd eventually confided in a teacher, who'd told the rest of the faculty.

Should I do something? Or should I ignore the rumours? Is it any of my business? While I have some idea of what goes on during these trips, any adult can fill in the blanks. I decided to act, but not as a nurse, as a parent, and I phoned Naomi's dad first.

'I think your daughter is going to have sex ...' is not the best way to start a conversation with a father. Instead, I asked if he was aware that his daughter was going away this weekend, which of course he was, and he wanted to know what the problem was. 'She's going with a group of boys, two girls and about twenty guys ...' I left the sentence unfinished, letting him fill in the blanks.

'Who the hell do you think you are ...' his tirade began. 'Are you saying I can't trust my daughter?'

'It's not about trust,' I wanted to say. It's about common sense. There's no way my parents would have let my sister go away with a bunch of boys at the age of fifteen. 'Are you calling me a bad father?'

I didn't tell him what I thought, instead I apologised. Time after time I have to remind myself not to impose my values on others. But surely any father, in any part of the world, would feel the same as me. Because of those harsh words I did not call Corinne's parents for fear of any repercussions.

The following Wednesday, Naomi and Corinne were standing in my office, bawling their eyes out.

The weekend had gone according to plan, for Naomi at least. She'd spent the night in Luke's hotel room. But things had not gone to plan for Corinne. Luke had booked another room for Corinne to stay in, with a male friend of his. 'He said it was the only room the hotel had left,' Corinne sobbed, 'he said it would be OK.' Corinne had been forced to spend the night with Luke's friend, a stranger to her. She was trying to figure out if she'd been raped.

Corinne was confused because she had agreed (reluctantly) to sharing the room and hence the bed. She couldn't remember exactly how or when she had consented to sex because she'd had 'a bit to drink' but she was sure she never really wanted to but felt like she 'had no choice'.

The school counsellor, doctor and the rest of the nursing staff became involved in helping Corinne and Naomi work through this problem, and thankfully, Corinne eventually came to the conclusion that she had not been raped but that she had made a mistake and panicked. In France, the age of consent is fifteen years old, making them both of legal consenting age, and the boys only a year or two older. Regardless of this, your first experience shouldn't leave you wondering if you've been raped.

Naomi also ended up seeing the counsellor. She felt guilty, and resented Luke for his part in what had happened. It's not the way anyone dreams their first time will be, but I wonder if anyone's first time works out the way they imagine.

Retelling and writing this story down hurts for me – I had tried to do what I felt was right. But by thinking like a father, I'd overstepped the line as a nurse and been attacked for caring. But I'd do it again.

A change of legislation since this incident means that I'm legally not allowed to call the parents now. Naomi's father didn't want my input before when I had the chance to warn him, but I bet he'd beg to hear what I have to say now if he had any inkling of what went on.

Not calling Corinne's family before the trip remains one of my biggest career regrets. I'd been intimidated by the reaction of Naomi's father. Perhaps Corinne's parents would have listened.

Dilemma

As you can see with the events surrounding Corinne and Naomi, confidentiality is not black and white; in fact it's very much a murky shade of grey.

It had seemed harmless fun at first, well, harmless to Sheryl and the rest of the kids she hung out with. But there are two types of pleasures in life: those that are free, and those that you have to pay for (in one way or another). And, this time, it was Sheryl's time to pay.

'Can I see a female nurse?' Sheryl asked. I didn't question why, but she felt the need to explain anyway. 'It's a girl problem.' If a seventeen-year-old girl wants to see a female nurse, then I'm happy to oblige.

I ushered Sheryl into Michaela's office and let them be.

What girl doesn't love attention? Sheryl wasn't picky in the sort of attention she got, and boys knew this about her and tried their luck. I had heard rumours that many home runs were scored, but from the look on Michaela's face when Sheryl had left her office, I had the sinking feeling that a lot of those boys weren't going to be feeling lucky for much longer.

'What a mess,' Michaela exclaimed once we were alone and I dutifully asked what was wrong.

Sheryl needed to see a gynaecologist because her 'girl's problem' was a very nasty case of genital warts that had become painful.

'I never knew they could get painful,' Michaela admitted, 'so I said we'd get an appointment urgently.'

After three months in a London walk-in STD clinic I'd seen more penises than I care to remember; small, big, crooked, two-toned, squishy, bendy, deadly, and one that rested just above the knee, but I couldn't remember a case of painful warts, although that was probably because I only dealt with male patients. I could imagine that friction (from a lot of sex) combined with large warts could lead to inflammation, and perhaps bleeding, or create the perfect environment for a bacterial infection.

Sheryl saw the gynaecologist the following day. It meant a thirty-minute trip to the hospital, but she was desperate to go as soon as possible, and was treated for an acute bacterial infection, after which she would eventually begin treatment for the genital warts. In the meantime she was not to have sex until her symptoms had resolved, and even then she had to use a condom, to offer some protection to others.

Teenagers don't do abstinence well, and understand STDs even less. I was reminded of a young couple, Camilla and Mark, who had recently fallen in love and become first-time lovers. Camilla then found out she might have Hepatitis A; she had told her boyfriend about this, and he had said it didn't bother him because he 'loved' her. It was a huge relief when her blood tests came back clear, but it was a scary reminder of the way young people don't fully understand the implications of such a diagnosis, and how powerful (or blinding) first love can be.

Sheryl put us in a very difficult position. She was seen around campus with a new man on her arm, a young student called Paul.

What would you do if you saw someone with an infectious disease potentially about to have intimate contact with a young man?

I'd never come across such a situation before and I turned to my colleagues and Dr Fritz for advice. It turns out we could not tell possible partners what she had as it was non-life threatening and confidentiality was the ultimate winner.

But we had to do something.

In the end, Michaela spent an hour talking to Sheryl, who promised she would try not to have sex, but if something did happen, she would inform her partner before intercourse and use a condom. It wasn't ideal, but it was the best we could do.

We also began a series of talks to small groups of students in their dorms.

The message was: 'There are STDs at this school.' I always stress this because some students think I'm kidding. Eye contact works well: 'You could have one.' I enjoy the reaction as everyone leans away from the person I'm staring out, and then I engage another: 'Or you could have one and not even know it.'

The message is simple: STDs are in our school. They always have been, and always will be – and they can happen to anyone.

CHAPTER THREE

School Nursing

Itch

School nursing isn't all about sex, and you must remember, I've been here ten years, and it's easy to remember the most shocking or interesting cases. In reality, much of my job revolves around much more mundane problems. But the thing is, nothing ever ends up being 'mundane' when you're dealing with children …

At all costs we wanted to avoid mass hysteria, but these things nearly always get out. Confidentiality is such a fickle thing at times, especially when teenagers are involved, especially when teenage *girls* are involved.

Tracy sat in my office, head bent forward, while I combed through her hair with my gloved fingers.

'Do I have them?' she asked. She certainly did have 'them', and as harmless as head lice are, there's no easy way to tell a girl she is infested.

'You've got the biggest nits I've ever seen,' I confessed, and she let out a brief scream of horror.

'They come in different sizes?'

'It seems they do, I've never seen such monsters, nor so many,' I joked, trying to make light of the situation. Tracy let out another gasp, then begged me to get rid of them and not say a word. 'No one can know. Please don't tell anyone.'

I reassured her that head lice were perfectly common in schools and completely harmless. I said I wouldn't tell anyone, but added that we would have to check her roommate as well as washing all her bedding and clothes. 'It's hard to keep something like this quiet, but don't worry, you're probably not the first and definitely not the only one.'

There's comfort in sharing an affliction, like a common cold or head lice, as long as it's something harmless. Knowing that you're not alone in your suffering somehow makes the burden easier … that is, so long as you're not the one accused of being the source of the outbreak. But judging by how well established the infestation was in Tracy's hair, it would be fair to assume she was the original source. I of course refrained from telling her.

The following morning twenty or so girls stormed the health centre, led by their spokeswoman, Anastasia. 'You have to give us shampoo,' she declared. She also insisted on being told who the source of the head lice outbreak was. At sixteen years of age, Anastasia was already a princess, not in name, but by her demanding behaviour. When you have someone to blame, it's easier to accept your condition because it wasn't *you* that is dirty or has bad hygiene habits, although the girls didn't realise cleanliness often has nothing to do with head lice. Despite my pleas that no one was to blame, and explaining that any one of them could be the source of any infestation they wouldn't relent and would not move until they each received shampoo and combs.

'I'll need to take a look at your head first,' I said, but Anastasia insisted that they get shampoo regardless if they had lice or not. 'No one is leaving until we get some.' Anastasia was a particularly headstrong student and she stood firm, with her arms crossed, feet apart, refusing to budge. The rest of the group followed her lead and stayed put.

'If you'll let me take a look, it won't take long to find out if you're infected, then I can order some.' I didn't have twenty bottles of shampoo, or twenty nit combs, and the local pharmacy would have to put in a special order to get enough, which would take another 24 hours. But Anastasia's argument was that it didn't matter if she had them or not, because she wouldn't feel 'clean' until she got treatment and she wanted to be 100 per cent sure. 'I won't sleep knowing someone in the dorm has lice,' she declared.

I tried to reassure her. 'Have you been scratching?' I asked. She said 'no' but everyone suddenly began to itch their scalp; I had to resist the urge to scratch my own.

'I bet it's Tracy,' said a voice from the back.

'Yeah, she's not here, she's always got dirty hair,' added Anastasia.

The witch-hunt had begun. I had to put a stop to it before people and reputations got hurt. I asked Anastasia if she kept her hair nice and clean. 'I shampoo every day. I always have clean hair.'

'Actually, head lice love clean hair.' There were gasps of shock.

'That isn't funny,' replied Anastasia.

'Who's trying to be funny?'

Head lice don't actually wander around in search of clean hair, or think to themselves 'here's a nice clean person to infect', they just find it easier to attach to clean hair, and find it a bit harder to stick to greasy hair.

'Perhaps you are infected, maybe you're the source.' I took a step away from Anastasia, and the rest of the girls looked at her as if she'd announced she had leprosy.

'No way, there's no way I'm the source. I'm not even itching.'

'Then you won't mind me having a look to make sure.' She realised she had trapped herself, and to prove she was 'clean' she agreed to sit down and let me comb through her hair, while everyone watched.

She was clean, but none of the other girls wanted to be checked, at least not in such a public forum, and over the day, they trickled in to be seen one by one. There were six more cases picked up, although none as severe as Tracy's. No one ever found out she was the probable source, and within two weeks everyone was in the clear, and the crisis soon behind them.

Head lice crop up once or twice every year, although one year, the junior boys' dorm had a constant stream of cases. It wasn't until we checked the dorm parents that we discovered the source. They felt incredibly guilty, but it helps people when I tell them that even my children, the sons of a nurse, have had them; my wife doesn't know I share such details, but it's too late now.

Sores

The nits were forgotten, but they'd be back. They always come back, along with other common bugs, viruses, funguses and bacteria. It can't be avoided when you've got six dorms packed with 50–80 kids, with 2–4 kids per room. It doesn't help when the kids share everything, from their drinks, lips, and more intimate bits … lots more of which later. Right now I was faced with a new problem, a common one … and something I'd never seen before.

Rebecca, aka Becks, had what looked like a pimple. As pimples go, it was a healthy specimen. It was a lovely size with a ripe yellow head that was pleading to be squeezed. But it wasn't where it should be, where everyone can see, in the centre of her face, but on her thigh.

'Should I pop it?' she asked, and I wanted to say 'Yes, let me do it', but that's the wrong thing to do. Squeezing such delectable treats can make the infection worse, as well as help it spread.

'No,' I said, and she looked as disappointed as I sounded. 'Just leave it alone, and it'll go away in a few days.'

The next day another pimple had appeared, a close neighbour.

'I told you not to pop it.' The first pimple was just a yellow crust now, while the second was coming along nicely.

'I didn't. I bumped it on something,' she protested. 'Are you sure it's a pimple though? I never get pimples.' Judging by the porcelain smooth skin on her face, no pimple would be brave enough to blemish such perfection, but pimples on the legs could be a random event, or not.

'An infected hair perhaps,' I suggested and she sighed, a wry smile on her lips. 'Do you see any hairs on my legs?'

She didn't have hairy legs. 'You don't even have stubble,' I remarked, and she sat there shaking her head in sadness at my ignorance. Teenage girls, especially older teenage girls, have perfect skin and non-hairy legs. A bit different from girls in my school days, although that may be a local trait of women from the deep south of New Zealand.

I digress.

Two pimples on a thigh is not a crisis, and the bursting of the first could explain the appearance of the second. 'Leave them alone, wash with soap and water, dry gently, and I'll see you on Monday.'

Lots can happen over a weekend, and on Monday morning Becks had a dozen pimples scattered over her left thigh, with two on the right.

'They're not pimples.' Rebecca was worried. 'They keep on spreading. Is it something contagious?' Simple acne is not contagious, but this was something more. I turned to my colleague Michaela for advice.

'It's a strange place to get pimples, what do you think it is?'

She knew straight away what it was. 'You've never seen school sores before?' she said incredulously. I shook my head. I had seen school sores, but had never actually seen anyone with it in such a place. I'd only ever seen it around the mouth and nose. 'Although it is an unusual place to get it,' she added, almost as if in apology.

School sores, also commonly called impetigo, is a common bacterial skin infection caused by the staphylococcus or streptococcus bacterium. This bacterium is very common and most of us carry it on our skin, but it can get into a cut or break in the skin and cause an infection. It is very contagious. It can be passed by direct skin-to-skin contact, or sharing towels, and we see it with a lot of children, although often on the face, around the lips. But it's not an emergency, and I'd never seen it before in the emergency room, or even in a general ward.

But that's because these illnesses aren't usually life threatening, and will rarely make it to the emergency room, and your local GP or even practice nurse can treat. By the time Becks saw Dr Fritz the sores had spread onto her lower back and calves. In this case he prescribed an oral antibiotic over a topical antibiotic cream because he felt the infection more systemic. Within a week the sores were gone.

The real deal

Not all rashes, blemishes or spots are created equal. I felt sorry for Diego because he looked worse than I ever had, and that's quite the accomplishment. I had some pretty serious acne in my adolescence, but Diego's face broke the record books for the number of spots per square inch of skin; even his pimples had pimples. The worst thing of all was that scars were beginning to form. I wanted to help, and knew of a method which had worked wonders for every patient I'd recommended it to. I never expected my good intentions to go wrong.

People say spots are 'harmless' and 'just part of being a teenager', but they're so much more. Acne has a direct impact on your social life. Teenagers can be so cruel. No matter how beautiful you are on the inside, for the treacherous years, it's so often what's on the outside that is what matters first.

'Mum said I'd grow out of it.' Diego was sitting in my office at my request because I was trying to ascertain what he currently used to treat his skin, but more importantly how he felt about potentially being physically scarred for life. 'And Dad said I need to stop jerking off so much.' Diego managed a brief chuckle. 'But I've never had it this bad before.' His acne had become much worse since moving to boarding school, and he admitted that his parents had not seen him since it had worsened.

He'd tried various creams and facial washes, plus six months of an antibiotic called minocycline, but nothing really worked. He'd tried cutting out fried foods, junk food, and reluctantly admitted he'd even tried stopping masturbating, but only managed two nights without. He was the first and only teenager I'd met to ever admit going to such lengths. Such an admission told me far more than I needed to know, but did give me an indication of how serious he was about getting rid of his acne.

I felt good at being able to offer him a cure because it's not always easy to treat a chronic problem with a simple course of antibiotics. With bigger or more chronic problems we help people get through the acute stages of their illness, we help their asthma settle down or their heart to pump more effectively, but then we send them on their way, to live as best they can with their condition. I felt useful and glad that I would be able to solve his problem, and told him about Roaccutane.

Roaccutane, aka Isotretinoin, is brutally effective in the war on acne. It's so powerful that people taking it need to have monthly blood tests to check their liver and cholesterol levels. The course usually runs for about four months, of which the first two are uncomfortable if not downright painful.

During this time patients can expect their face to dry up, including their tear ducts, nasal and oral mucosa; their face looks almost stretched as the skin becomes parched. They say it's like their face is peeling off. People taking it have to avoid strong sunlight, and constantly have to apply moisturising lotion to their skin as it can sometimes break down and tear, especially around the mouth. To make matters even worse, patients can expect their acne to get worse within the first month. But every single subject I've met has been willing to make the sacrifice.

Such a vicious treatment needs to be prescribed and monitored by a doctor and it was the prescribing doctor's responsibility to inform the student what to expect. Dr Fritz focused on explaining the physical effects and if, after hearing how severe they could be, they still wanted to proceed, then treatment began as soon as we received written permission from a parent.

Diego leapt at the chance to finally get on top of his acne and his parents quickly agreed to the treatment. In their letter of consent, the parents agreed that they knew and understood the risks associated with Roaccutane, but what parent truly knows all the risks? For that matter, what nurse ever knows all the risks either?

By week two Diego's acne had become worse, and his parched, stretched skin looked like someone recovering from botched cosmetic surgery, as expected.

By week four his face was still stretched, although the acne was starting to improve.

By week six there was a marked improvement; there was still plenty of acne, but it was in full retreat, submerging back into the surrounding flesh, no longer angry or full of pus.

At eight weeks, another side effect became apparent. The end of term grades were out, and Diego's had dropped, a lot.

Students' grades oscillate up and down all the time, but significant drops, from an A average to a C average, are usually a symptom of something out of balance in the child's life. It may be due to physical reasons, like being sick, or some external influence. A noticeable drop in grade is often the first indicator of something serious.

'You never told me it causes depression.' Diego had come to the nurses' office and accused me of not informing him of the risks associated with Roaccutane. He'd been researching the drug online and had come across the psychological side effects, which neither the doctor nor I had mentioned. A bit of googling led him to an article clearly stating that in rare cases Roaccutane can cause depression or mood changes.

'I don't have the energy to care,' Diego told me – such succinct words to describe apathy of the mind – adding 'and I can't get out of bed.' No such thing exists as a teenager that leaps out of bed, bright and cheery, but those first words 'I don't have the energy to care' were worrying. I suggested that maybe he's just not getting enough sleep, or exercise, or a healthy diet.

'Nothing's changed, sir. It's the pills. All I want to do is sleep. I don't want to go to class. Even my friends keep asking me what's wrong. They say I'm not my normal self.'

If you look up any drug online and research its side effects, the list is endless, covering almost all possibilities. I researched the NHS guidelines for Roaccutane and got nearly one hundred side effects, from cataracts and seizures to pancreatitis, the latter of which tends to be life threatening. Regardless, it didn't stop me feeling guilty, and I told him I was sorry.

He stopped his treatment, and within a couple of weeks his mood improved, and by the middle of the following term his grades had returned to normal, as had his skin, although the acne didn't return quite as bad as before.

'I'd rather live with the pimples than be messed up the way that shit made me feel,' he said to me. 'I never want to feel that way again.'

I think it also helped that at this time he'd also found his first serious girlfriend, who could obviously see beneath the surface.

I'm now more cautious when recommending serious treatments, and while I have seen fantastic results when it's used properly, I make sure to mention the rare, but possible, psychological effects of Roaccutane as well. Though, perhaps most sadly, the majority of people are happier simply because they look good.

Parents' worst nightmare

Part one: Monique

Acne, communicable diseases, coughs, colds, rashes, cuts, grazes and bruises make up the bulk of my everyday work, but there are also less common problems. Fortunately these only come up once or twice a year. But once a year is enough, and it's every parent's worst nightmare.

Monique crashed. Lots of kids have a mini meltdown when they start studying International Baccalaureate, an advanced high school diploma that kids can choose to do in their last two years of school. Monique's problem was that she was only fifteen years old. She was in a class one year ahead of most people her age and naturally found it a little harder to fit in with the older kids. At least that's what I thought. Despite being slightly younger for her year, she did have two good friends from her hometown of Houston, so I wasn't worried overly much.

'I just need to sleep,' Monique confessed. Every student wants more sleep, it comes with being a teenager, but I was pleased Monique was at least being honest. Between the ages 12–16, most patients generally feel the need to justify coming to see the nurse, and will make up a whole barrage of symptoms to get excused from class. I appreciate honesty, and so I let Monique rest.

Monique was not a regular visitor to the health centre, but I saw her again the next day. 'I slept the whole night, but I still feel so tired,' Monique explained. 'And I feel a bit sick as well.' Yesterday I hadn't actually assessed her, as she wasn't unwell, and just wanted to rest. But I thought it worth finding out a bit more.

'Are you often so tired?'

'I guess so, but it seems worse this last month.'

'What do you mean exactly when you say you feel sick?' She had felt a bit nauseous for the last few days and put it down to being so exhausted. I checked her blood pressure, pulse and temperature – all normal. I also asked if she had ever had her iron levels checked. She didn't think so. I asked about her waterworks, bowels, appetite, and diet … I was trying to get as much information as possible to give me some idea of what could be going on.

It's not unusual to be unable to find a cause for a particular complaint or symptom, but what I can usually do is eliminate anything more serious. In this case, there was one last thing I had to ask.

'I have to ask a very personal question. There's no delicate way to put this, so I'll just say it. Is there any chance you could be pregnant?'

Monique vehemently denied the possibility. I let her rest for a couple of hours, after which she felt better and went back to class.

A week passed and I didn't see Monique at all, until I got a phone call from the local hospital. Three of our girls were in the local emergency room asking to see a doctor. One of them was Monique.

Confidentiality is paramount to any medical institution, but what's even more important is a patient's ability to pay. If you're not a European citizen then you pay for your privacy, and when Monique couldn't provide her insurance details, and had no way to pay for her treatment, the hospital called me.

'I'm so sorry.' Monique was sobbing over the phone. 'I just didn't know where to go. You can't tell my parents.' After calming her down I said I'd pick her and her friends up shortly. I really needed to know what was going on, but it had to be done in person, not over the phone, so I met the girls thirty minutes later in the hospital waiting room. Everyone was in tears.

'Please don't tell my parents, they'll kill me,' Monique pleaded as we began the drive back to school. Monique was pregnant, and she was trying to find somewhere she could get an abortion. 'I'm not going to tell them anything, Monique, not without your permission.' I did add that I would be talking with the other nurses and the school doctor. This issue was something I would need advice with, just as much as Monique.

'You're not going to tell my parents?' Monique was disbelieving until I explained that legally I wasn't able to.

'But perhaps your parents might surprise you. They might be more supportive than you think.'

'You obviously don't know who my dad is, do you?' I shook my head. 'He's a minister. He'll be furious because I'm pregnant, and he'd never forgive me because I tried to get an abortion. My life is over.' I couldn't think of anything useful to say, so after dropping the girls off with their dorm head I told Monique to come and see me in the morning after I'd had a chance to talk with the other nurses.

As a parent I would want to know if my child was pregnant, but ultimately the child needs someone safe to turn to. Monique had already put herself at risk by breaking out of the dorm at night-time. She had managed this by tying bed sheets together and climbing down the balcony from the third floor. This may look easy in the movies, but it's dangerous, let alone during the night, in winter, with ice and snow around. It could have been fatal.

I was still struggling with what to do. Normally I would advise the patient to tell her family, but the father's background certainly complicated things. I turned to my colleagues for advice.

'You're going to have to tell the parents,' said Michaela, 'otherwise this could get very, very messy.'

Meanwhile, Dr Fritz said we absolutely couldn't tell her parents, even though she was underage, because the child must have someone she can trust. 'We're not just legally bound; a patient's right to safe, unbiased care is at the core of any doctor's practice,' he explained.

I sometimes struggle with this law, and I can understand how parents get furious about it, but even underage children are legally entitled to confidentiality regarding their sexual health. Dr Fritz summed it up by adding that if children feel they have no one safe to turn to, they can put their life at risk. In this case, Monique and her friends could have died climbing out the window. Or, more worrying still, she could have turned to other, illegal, methods to terminate her pregnancy.

The other two nurses, the school's counsellor Cathy and I agreed to have a meeting with Monique. She brought along her closest friend, Alice, for support. 'I don't know what to do.' She was sobbing again. 'My parents will never forgive me for this.' She repeated those words, over and over, but when I suggested that there is nothing to forgive, she told me I was 'dreaming' and insisted she needed forgiveness. Michaela and Cathy tried to reassure her that there was nothing to forgive, but this only made her angry.

She needed forgiveness, at least in her mind, from her parents, maybe even from God, but most of all she would need to be able to forgive herself. 'Your parents might be more supportive than you think,' I kept suggesting, and she snorted in disgust at my continued ignorance. 'My dad is a minister. I'm not supposed to have sex outside of marriage. He'll hate me.'

'Your parents won't hate you,' I said, believing that I must be right. 'They will want to help you, be there for you.'

The truth is, you never know how a parent will react. All I had to go on was how I'd seen parents react in the hospital when I'd had to call them to say we had their child with us. It didn't matter if it was due to alcohol, drugs, self-harm, or even attempted home-abortions, the large majority of parents were relieved instead of angry.

Teenagers think a parent's anger is proportional to the problem created. A parent gets a little angry at their child who does not do their homework, and gets very angry when they find out their child has been in a fight at school, therefore a parent will be furious if they find out their daughter is pregnant.

This could be true, but the parents I've seen in these circumstances have been surprisingly supportive and relieved that they knew, and the children involved have been genuinely surprised to find their parents reacting in such a positive way. My line of questioning was with the purpose of trying to find out if Monique's parents were the supportive type, or the angry, yelling, make-the-situation-worse type.

I explained all this to Monique.

She asked for some time to think about it.

We saw her again the following morning. She'd made up her mind.

'I can't do this on my own,' she said.

Michaela was first to offer to be there for her. 'No matter what you decide, you won't be alone.'

Does that mean she doesn't want to be alone while she has an abortion? Or does that mean she doesn't want to make this decision alone and wants to tell her parents? I assumed the latter.

'Do you want me to call your mother?' I suggested. Just because mums are mums, and her daughter may become one, it seemed reasonable to make her the first person to tell.

'Yes, I'd like that. If you speak to her first.' Monique then began to cry. Michaela put her arms around her.

'It will all work out, it will be OK,' she crooned, gently stroking her hair as Monique buried her head in her chest.

Part two: the call

It doesn't get easier telling parents difficult news. Although, over time, I've developed a script to fall back on. I use the same opening line whatever the incident.

I've tried 'It's the hospital calling, we have your ...' which is OK, but it's not enough because you feel the panic rising already, the 'oh, no' or quickened breathing on the other end of the line. There's too much time to panic. Instead I start with 'Your daughter is fine, and well, but there is a serious matter I need to talk to you about.' I repeated those words to Monique's mother.

'Is she sick? Has there been an accident?' She was worried, but not panicked. 'Monique's fine, she's with me right now. Healthy and sound,' I added, my tone surprisingly light.

She asked what the problem was.

'She's very upset, and worried about telling you, but she wants to tell you herself.' I handed the phone to Monique and she burst into another round of tears.

'I'm sorry Mum, so sorry,' she pleaded. 'Please don't hate me.' I could hear her mother making soothing noises down the phone. 'Mum, I'm pregnant.' Michaela and I witnessed the relieved expression on Monique's face when she finished her call.

'They didn't yell at me,' was the first thing she said when the conversation ended. Her mother was flying out to meet her the next day. Monique left school and went home with her mother. She didn't come back to boarding school, although I do get the occasional message from her. She did have the baby and she seems to be happy, although I have no idea how much choice she had in her decision once she made the call to her parents, but she did make that choice, not me.

And what about the father of her child? It turned out he was a friend of a school friend, whom she'd met during a long weekend in Paris. There were many other students there; at least a couple of dozen staying at the five-star hotel her parents had booked her into. It had its own discotheque and like the rest of Europe, no one was fussy about age of consent. I don't know if he even knows he is a father, although we did encourage Monique to try and find a way of contacting him. I don't know that she ever did.

I learned a lot from my experience with Monique, but it will never be easy to tackle these situations. When all is said and done, we try to make decisions that are in the best interest of the patient. Things are never black and white, and each problem has its own unique solution. My opinion on abortion is irrelevant. I feel I helped Monique make her own decision, the decision that was best for her.

But I do worry. Often the parents of these children are not supportive, more restrictive, and it makes you wonder. If the children had more supportive and less absent parents would they ever find themselves in such serious situations feeling so alone?

Type I

Part one: the phobia

Roman was one of our regulars. It was his first time living away from home, and as far as fourteen-year-olds go, he was a good kid: quiet, hardworking with straight A grades to match, shy, yet not one to change his ways to suit others or fashion. He reminded me of myself at his age.

Since joining the school, Roman had dropped by the health centre almost every day just to 'touch base', as he called it. Half the time he was after something, usually for a minor problem, such as a scratchy throat or sniffly nose. Most times he left my office with nothing because after exchanging pleasantries, and having a chuckle over some mundane school gossip, he usually forgot what he came for and left content.

On this occasion, Roman had more than just a scratchy throat or tickly cough. This time Roman had spent the weekend alternating between two places; his bed and the toilet. When he was on the toilet he usually had a bucket between his legs. He was the tenth victim to fall foul of the diarrhoea and vomiting (D&V) bug – or Norovirus, as it has become known – over the last week and he would not be the last.

Apart from some simple medicines to hopefully ease the symptoms, there's not a lot you can do to help someone with a nasty case of gastroenteritis. Sometimes the medicines help with the nausea or the abdominal cramps, and sometimes they don't.

I'd checked on Roman several times over the weekend.

'Rest, small sips of fluid, and time,' I kept on reassuring him.

'Nothing helps. You must have something else, anything.' Roman was pleading for medication, but so far none of them were making much difference. Fortunately by Sunday morning his symptoms had improved, but he was still miserable. By Sunday night his appetite had not returned but he was tolerating fluid fine without having to run to the toilet after every mouthful.

By Monday morning his diarrhoea, cramps, vomiting and nausea had stopped and he managed some toast without any ill effects, although he still looked pale and parched. I kept him in the health centre to build up his strength and make sure he drank enough.

By Tuesday he was eating normally, but something didn't look quite right. 'Are you sure you're drinking enough?' I asked, noting his still dry lips.

'I'm drinking plenty,' he insisted.

I asked exactly how much and he insisted he had drunk three litres of water in the last 24 hours. 'I'm fine, just a bit dry. I can't afford to miss any more classes or I'm going to get too far behind.'

I let him go to class.

'We've missed you,' I said when I next saw Roman. It was Friday and I had missed his daily visits.

'Too much work to catch up on,' he explained.

'You back to normal?' I asked.

'Pretty much,' he replied, but I wasn't convinced. He looked pale and still had dry lips, and I told him so.

'I'm drinking heaps, but I just can't get enough. I'm constantly thirsty.' At those words, I became very worried. I asked Roman if I could do a blood test.

'I don't like needles,' he replied.

No one 'likes' needles, especially teenagers. During the winter season we give mass flu vaccinations and after receiving parental consent, get permission for about three-quarters of the students; we usually end up injecting about 300 students in the course of a morning. The girls feed off each other with their hysteria (though, for 299 of them the hysteria is part of the show; it's not a real phobia). As for the boys, they're not as loud, they try to hide it, but they're frightened as well.

'On the count of three,' I usually say and inject them on the count of one. Both boys and girls seem disappointed when the injection is over before they realise it's been given. The majority of them admit that it didn't hurt.

I explained all this to Roman.

'There's no way you're coming anywhere near me with a needle,' Roman insisted. 'Can't you do another test? What do you want to look for anyway?'

I didn't want to cause unnecessary worry, but I had to stress how important the test was.

'I want to assess your blood sugar.' Roman had no idea what this meant. 'I really have to do this test. It's just a tiny prick on the end of your finger. It won't hurt.' A tear slid down Roman's right cheek and his voice cracked. 'I can't take needles, I just can't. You don't understand. Can't you do it another way, please.' Roman's arms and legs began to shake slightly, a side effect from the nervous release of adrenaline.

Without the slightest doubt I knew Roman was that one out of 300 that had a true phobia of needles. I desperately hoped my blood test would allay my fears.

It took twenty minutes for Roman to prepare himself before we eventually got a blood sample. The result was bad. His blood sugar was very high. Roman had developed diabetes.

Part two: the outcome

Diabetes is divided into two main categories, Type I and Type II. Type II is the most common. It develops as a result of lifestyle, such as being overweight, lack of exercise, poor diet and so on. The cells responsible for controlling blood sugar become less responsive, or can't produce enough insulin. People can improve their condition through improving the above risk factors.

Type I happens suddenly and can happen to anyone at any time. Your own immune system suddenly decides to attack your own body. For some reason it identifies the cells that are responsible for producing insulin as the enemy, and goes about destroying those cells. It's the more serious of the two because there is no solution. Type I sufferers need injections of insulin for the rest of their life.

In both types of diabetes, good control is vital. For Type I diabetes, good control is not only essential for staying alive, if practised from a young age, it can reduce the impacts of the disease in later life.

The immediate danger is low blood sugar or 'hypo', a highly dangerous event as you can lose consciousness and eventually die due to brain damage. High blood sugar can also be dangerous, making your blood turn to acid.

If you manage to avoid excessive highs and lows, a reasonably well-controlled diabetic can still suffer long-term side effects – even if their blood sugars are only a little high. It may take 10–20 years to see the results, but the effects of slightly raised blood sugar over a long period of time are permanent; damaged blood vessels, poor circulation to the limbs, blindness. It's not uncommon for Type 1 diabetics to have a lower limb amputated.

Roman had developed Type I diabetes.

While I've looked after many patients in hospital with both types I and II, Roman was the second person I had ever seen develop the disease from scratch. It was new to me and life changing for Roman, but this wasn't the time to frighten him with all the details. He was terrified already, and with his genuine phobia of needles, Roman was in for the most difficult time of his young life. Diabetes, hospitals and needles all go hand in hand. It cannot be avoided.

I can remember the absolute terror on Roman's face the first day of his stay in hospital as he grabbed my shirt, pleading, tears coursing down his face. 'Don't leave me. Don't let them do this to me.' I sat beside him clasping his hand as he begged. 'You have to stop them, please, there has to be another way.'

I felt close to tears myself; I wanted nothing more than to stop the needles, the intravenous lines and the infusions, but I needed to stay strong for him.

'I'm sorry' – I found myself saying that a lot over the next few hours – 'but there is no other way.' Roman's sobs swelled, but he held out his arm. I was relieved when the doctor got the line in first go – it's not always so easy when the pressure is on, and I felt certain that if he missed, I really would have to restrain Roman. I felt helpless that I couldn't do more, and it was painful to watch him suffer. I had to hold him, a hold that felt almost like a restraint, while the doctor did what had to be done, to save his life.

Roman spent one week in hospital before he was discharged. His mother came to stay with him for the next month while he adjusted to his new life.

After daily meetings with Roman's mother and daily monitoring of his blood sugars, we had a decision to make; what to do with Roman.

'Can you look after my son?' his mother asked. Michaela, Justine and I looked at each other, wondering who was going to deal with this loaded question.

'We can look after him,' Michaela began, 'but we're not sure if this is the best environment.'

'You're all trained nurses,' countered his mother. This didn't feel like a meeting. She wanted concrete answers. 'Can you look after him or not?'

'Well, yes we can, but we can't watch him 24 hours a day. He'll be sleeping in a dorm, with other kids and teachers who don't know about diabetes,' Michaela said.

'I can't watch him 24 hours a day either,' Roman's mother said. 'What's the difference with him being here or at home? I don't see a problem.' There was silence.

I did see a problem. It wasn't just about supervision, it was about developing good habits that would impact the rest of Roman's life. What he learned now and what practices he developed to control his blood sugars would determine his life expectancy.

On top of his medical needs, which included everything from managing his diet, recognising a hypo and knowing what to do, the education side of things was a major task, and would affect his future.

To top it off, he had the worst needle phobia I'd ever seen.

I informed his mother of these factors, in detail.

'But you're a nurse, isn't this part of your job?' was her response.

Many parents are not easy to deal with; they don't always react the way you expect them to, especially when it comes to accepting professional opinions. I try to avoid giving parental advice for a variety of reasons, not least because I don't always find the right words to express myself.

Sometimes problems are so unique, so rare, that the right way to handle things is not clear. I'm not sure if that's a reflection of my own insecurities, or an intrinsic part of school nursing.

He's got a life changing diagnosis that he's going to have to deal with every single day of his life. He needs to be at home, and he needs to be with his family. How could she not understand this?

I wasn't getting through to Roman's mother, and I had to take control of my own emotions because I couldn't understand why a parent would not want their son at home.

I didn't do very well. I had to speak my mind.

'If he were my child, I'd have him at home. He needs his mum and dad. We can manage him here, but we can't provide the same level of support that you as parents can. We have 400 children here to monitor. My advice is to take your son home.'

My honesty was greeted with silence.

'I'm sorry, but it's the truth,' I was blabbing now to fill the void.

Finally she spoke. 'That's not very professional,' she said, her voice icy calm. I thought speaking as one parent to another that she would appreciate my straightforward opinion. I felt angry. Surely I'd done the right thing speaking the truth, but Justine, who had been quiet all along, decided to butt in.

'He's speaking as a parent, not a nurse, I'm sorry …' Justine began, but I cut her off.

'I'm sorry you're upset, but no one else is going to say this to you – you need to take your son home. He needs you, he needs his mother.' My words infuriated her, and she asked me to leave the room while she talked to the other two nurses. To keep the peace I left, but I found myself pleading with her first: 'My job as a nurse is to give you the whole picture, that's all I'm trying to do.'

Was I really just trying to give her the whole picture, or was I judging her? What was my role? Was I a nurse? A parent? I was both, but I'm supposed to be a professional and separate the two. However, when you live and care for the kids in your school, it doesn't always seem possible to do this. I knew that if Roman stayed at school, he would not get the attention he needed.

He needed someone, a nurse or a parent, who could be there when problems arose, because here, I've got 399 other children to take care of. We could advise him what to eat, but not be there to make sure he ate it, let alone weighed his food. We could remind him to check his sugar before bed, and to have a snack to get him through the night, but we weren't going to be there to make sure.

We weren't going to be there in the night if he woke up confused because his blood sugar was low. We wouldn't be there to tell him to stay in his bunk bed, while we fetch something sugary. What if he fell from his bunk in a confused state? It wasn't safe for him at the school.

I spoke out because we can't provide what a home can provide. Someone to be there when he needs someone most.

Roman stayed till the end of the year before changing boarding schools. His blood sugars were a disaster, his understanding of the disease unhealthy, he had more than his share of close calls. We were lucky he made it to the end of the year without serious harm. Sadly Roman couldn't see this – but what can you expect of a kid who's had a life changing diagnosis? It's why I felt so strongly he needed to be at home.

Roman went to university and he regularly 'touches base' with me. He still thanks me for being there during his darkest moments, and tells me 'you're one of the good guys'. I've never told him about my outburst with his mother. I just ask him what his HBA1C is.

This is a blood test that gives an overall indicator of his diabetes control. His reply is usually, 'could be better'.

I don't blame his mother for how things turned out. I don't blame anyone, although when I relate this story, I still get a little upset that his mother attacked me for suggesting he be taken home. I just can't understand that.

It seems I'm regularly overstepping my role, but then that's what school nurses do when they think they're doing the best for their patients, when they care so much for them. We want to make sure everyone sees the whole picture, from as broad a perspective as possible. We'll disagree with the doctor, argue our cause and speak up for those who are too scared to speak up for themselves.

Gravity

On average once every two months I'm given a reminder of the nature of gravity, although the speed with which Eva hit the floor was actually faster than the speed of that force.

To hit the ground as fast as she did, she had to actually throw herself at the ground. To this day, and after twenty years of nursing, I had never seen anyone hit the ground so fast, and with no warning. The odd thing about her landing was that she was lying nicely on her side, with her hair splayed out beautifully around her face, her body conveniently lying in the recovery position. I wasn't convinced. Her head hadn't even made a 'thunk' when it came in contact with the floor.

To the average non-medical person, this is a frightening scene. To me, it's usually nothing to worry about.

'Eva, can you hear me?' There was no reaction. While I tried to rouse her with my voice, I felt her pulse and looked at her breathing. All were within normal limits. After the verbal stimulation begins the physical stuff, like gently shaking the shoulders, or grasping and squeezing the hand. When this doesn't work, the normal procedure is to apply increasing levels of pain, to determine to what degree she is actually unconscious.

I liked Eva, and as I didn't actually want to hurt her, I did what

I always do when I see a suspicious faint. I called out to the other nurses: 'Can you bring me a needle, I need to test her pain threshold.' This had the desired result and there was a brief stirring from Eva. Of course she couldn't wake up straight away, as that wouldn't look normal, at least in her eyes. If only she knew that nothing about this situation was normal.

I could have checked her blood pressure, or even her blood sugar, but the needle test is much more effective.

Michaela handed me a needle. 'I'm just going to insert it under your fingernail,' I explained as I took a firm grasp of Eva's hand. She began to make moaning noises and pulled her hand away before bolting upright. Her 'symptoms' magically had disappeared.

Just for the record, I never use needles when assessing unconsciousness. I do administer pain, as it is allowed, but not in this manner and not in this situation. This was just to let Eva know that I was in charge of the situation.

It would be a big mistake to assume Eva was just faking it, even though I felt without any doubt she was. The time you decide to assume, without doing a check-up, is the time you get it wrong. Once I had Eva sitting in my office feeling 'unwell', I checked her blood pressure, pulse, neurological observations, and even her blood sugar, which were completely normal.

After half an hour of monitoring, and a note from the health centre excusing her from skiing for the afternoon, she left my office, practically skipping down the corridor.

Only a handful of students are so dramatic, although it's this very drama that makes it so suspicious. But that's just part of the job – giving a teenage girl a credible escape from a bizarre and ultimately exaggerated situation. It always make me wonder – what on earth must be going through their minds in the moments before they decide to faint or pretend to be ill?

Breathless

I've seen it drive some nurses to drink, change placements, or even leave nursing altogether. When you're at home, and the dribble of a late autumn sun punctured by towering peaks sinks out of sight, and you're desperate for sleep, the last thing you want is the emergency phone to ring. You never know what you're going to get, minor or traumatic, harmless or frightening.

Three nights of my week are spent on call, all afternoon, evening, and through the night. Call-outs can be anything, anytime, anywhere. It's usually just a kid that's been sick. 'I don't want to catch it!' I feel like saying to the house parent on the other end of the line. That, or 'give them a bucket.'

It's not the dorm parent's fault; sometimes they're new to the job, and new to being a guardian *in loco parentis*. (The Mexican students told me that 'loco' means crazy, which suits me fine.)

It was late Saturday night and my pyjamas were pulling me to bed when the phone rang.

'Mourad can't breathe, call an ambulance, he can't breathe,' cried Mrs Patton, her voice quivering with panic. I've heard this many times, mainly in hospital, where it's generally been true – out here it usually isn't. But you never know, and that's what drives nurses insane. You don't know what you're going to find. Luckily, I could hear my patient's loud breathing in the background. Whatever was wrong, he wasn't having trouble breathing, quite the opposite. I'd heard this sort of breathing plenty of times before and had a good idea of what was going on.

I told Mrs Patton I'd be right there, and to not call an ambulance just yet.

That's a big call to make. If I was wrong, time would be of the essence, but I felt 99 per cent sure my suspicion would be confirmed.

I found Mourad in the centre of the dorm, lying on his back on the floor, a crowd of onlookers making him worse. Apart from his rapid breathing, which was at least 100 breaths per minute, his hands were curled inwards, and his eyes were rolling around wildly.

Mourad was having a panic attack.

They're terrifying to watch. The patient barely responds to you, they lie staring at the ceiling, or rolling their eyes back into their skull, sometimes clutching their chest; 'h … h … hurts' they manage, or 'c … c … c … can't … bre … bre … breathe'. But it's harmless, self-limiting, and some people say just wait it out.

'He needs to go to hospital.'

'He needs oxygen.'

'It's his heart, he's having a heart attack.'

Crowds never help, so I ordered everyone out the room.

Mrs Patton leapt into action to gather up the children, but Mohammad, Mourad's roommate wanted to stay.

'I'm family,' he said, 'his dad wants me to stay.' I had no problem with one person staying, a friend, a family member, although I was worried about his dad being informed already.

I knelt on the floor, grabbed Mourad's hand and started to talk, calmly, slowly, reassuring him he'd be fine. He didn't see me at first, but after a couple of minutes something got through, and his eyes acknowledged me, and his breathing began to slow.

'Can you hear me?' He managed a nod. 'I'm going to give you some medicine. Would you like that?' Another nod.

For instances like these, we have an agreement with Dr Fritz to give a relaxant, Lorazepam. It's a benzodiazepine, and they've been around a long time, and work very well. I placed the tablet under his tongue and within ten minutes his breathing had slowed even further.

Thirty minutes later he was breathing normally, lying in his own bed and able to talk. Mohammad was sitting next to him, reading from the Koran.

'He said it helps,' Mohammad explained. 'I'll sit with him all night, it's not a problem.' Mohammad was a true friend.

Another call came in – it was time to talk to Mourad's father.

'He has to go to hospital.' His words were not angry, but desperate, a loving father stranded apart, both in distance and worry at this confusing illness.

'He's going to be fine' didn't work, and neither did explaining about a 'panic attack'. Mourad's father became insistent.

'How do you know it's not his heart, he's never been sick like this.'

It's hard to explain that something so dramatic is harmless, but as a nurse I have to do what is right for the patient, not the parent. The worst thing I could do now, at midnight, was to bundle Mourad into a car and take the forty-minute journey to hospital. They'd make him wait. It wouldn't be deliberate; that's just the triage system. The nurse would see a sleepy but well boy, not in need of urgent treatment. We could spend hours in the waiting room, that's what happens on a Saturday night. I told his father all of this.

'He has to go.' I couldn't get through his fear. 'I demand it, he's my son, and you have to take care of my flesh and blood.'

I was torn between the father's agony and what I knew to be in the best interest of my patient. I hoped he would understand in the morning. I said 'sorry' as I hung up the phone.

Mourad woke the next morning as if nothing had happened. He got up, got dressed, and went to breakfast. He spoke to his father, and I took him to see Dr Fritz, who recommended professional counselling. Thankfully, his father was no longer angry at me, and I never was with him.

Mourad had two more attacks that year, before he was withdrawn from school.

'He's homesick,' his father said. 'He doesn't like living away from home.'

And he was probably right in his diagnosis. I suspect Mourad's problem stopped once he got home.

I see about a dozen panic attacks each year. They can come out of the blue, but once one's happened, it's not unusual for a repeat; it's why doctors recommend counselling from the very first episode.

Doing the right thing against a parent's wishes is frightening as you really have to be sure about your diagnosis and your treatment. Dr Fritz always backs us up, but that's because we trust each other's judgment, as well as being comfortable asking questions when we're unsure.

Francesca

My role as a school nurse is sometimes harder than anything I've done before. It's not the isolation, the being on call in the middle of the night for emergencies, or even the vast scope of injuries and illness that I see. Sometimes the hardest thing about this job is trying to keep my charges safe from their own family, especially when money is involved; there are times when people think the more money they spend, the better the outcome, no matter how they behave.

Take Francesca. Francesca was a petite Sicilian girl who was captain of the volleyball team, the lead actor in several of the school plays, chairman of the school social committee as well as being on the school ski team, and an all-around nice kid. As the years went by, she began to slow down.

'I've got so much work to do, I just don't have the time,' was her explanation as to why she wasn't trying out for the upcoming theatre production. She had played a major part in the last three and it had come as a surprise to everyone, especially her drama teacher, but it's not unusual for students to drop some extra-curricular activities, even when it's their passion, when they reach their senior year. The workload is impressive and if you want to do well, then like most things in life, you have to focus and sacrifice.

I didn't know that she was no longer on the social committee, although if I had, it still wouldn't have given me reason to be concerned. But when she said she wasn't going to play volleyball this year I did suggest this was a bad idea. 'You need to exercise your body, not just your mind,' I told her, and she managed a smile.

'Heard that line a few dozen times,' she replied, 'but I'm just too tired.' Every single student complains of being tired, so I didn't find it necessary to find out more this time.

A few days before the Christmas break I was called to see Francesca in her room. Her roommate, Angela had called the emergency number because Francesca had fallen over getting out the shower, and wouldn't get up. I've had a few close calls when entering the girls' dorm, especially in the evening when they're in various states of undress and have decided to visit their neighbours. I normally get one of the dorm staff to chaperone me, but they were all busy that evening.

'I'm coming in,' I called out at the entrance to the girls' dorm, 'is it safe to?' 'Of course it's safe.' Angela greeted me in the corridor and led me to her room. 'Is it safe to come in? Is everyone decent?' I called out again, before entering the room, 'the nurse is here.' Angela opened the door and ushered me inside. Francesca had moved from the floor and was lying in bed, the covers up to her neck, her face pale, her eyes half closed. I sat on the side of her bed to check her pulse, blood pressure, temperature and breathing.

'I didn't really faint,' were the first words out of her mouth. 'I just felt so weak, so tired, I didn't have the strength to stand. I just sat down.'

Her blood pressure was a touch on the low side, 95/70, but I wasn't too worried. A normal adult BP is about 120/80, but in nearly all the teenage girls I see, it's usually around 100–105/70–80, and Francesca was a very slight young woman.

'I didn't fall,' she insisted. 'I'm just so tired'. Her pulse was fine, and she claimed to be otherwise well, but a healthy young girl should not be collapsing from exhaustion.

I could think of a dozen reasons she might feel this way; I needed to find out more.

I began with the usual questions: Did she skip meals? Was she getting enough sleep? Did she stay up late studying? Was she working out at the gym too much?

She said she didn't skip meals, she did get enough sleep, didn't stay up late studying, and had stopped all her sports because she didn't have the strength, but the pieces of the puzzle fell into place when she said she'd been vegetarian her whole life. Further questioning revealed a very heavy menstrual cycle, as well as a lot of pain.

You've possibly come to the same conclusion I have. I took her to the doctor the following morning for a blood test to confirm my suspicions. However, holidays intervened. Francesca didn't get to see her blood results before leaving for the Christmas break, and when she came back she had her own doctor's report.

'He's one of the top doctors in the country,' Francesca explained, handing me a prescription to fill. 'Can you get it here?'

She was diagnosed with Somatoform Autonomic Dysfunction and prescribed the following:

- Ceraxon injections, daily for one month
- Actovegin injections, daily for one month
- Glycine tablets
- Semax nasal spray
- Riboksin tablets
- Magnesium tablets

I had to google what the disease was, as well as most of the medications.

'Have you started treatment?' I asked, hoping she had not. She shook her head. I then showed her the blood results from our recent test, which indicated she was severely anaemic.

She agreed to go to see Dr Fritz with me, whereupon she was advised not to take the treatment from the Sicilian doctor, and instead began a course of intravenous injections of iron.

Within one month Francesca was a different person. It's amazing what a bit of iron does. I see many adolescent girls with low iron, and I wish I had picked up on Francesca's problem sooner, although I am relieved that we were able to intervene before she started her bizarre treatment plan from her home doctor.

Dr Fritz spent the following few days investigating the medications prescribed, and came to the conclusion that the injections were not only unnecessary, but in fact harmful, banned in most places, and could have caused a lot of problems.

I can't think of another role where I'm constantly second-guessing every medical certificate I see. The problem is not Sicilian doctors, or Russian doctors, or doctors from wherever – it doesn't matter where they're from as every place has good and bad medical 'professionals'. The problem is parents who think spending a fortune means better care, or parents looking for treatment to suit their personal diagnosis.

Some of the more memorable prescriptions I've seen in my time are:

Thyroxine for a student with a normal thyroid. We became suspicious when we discovered her wearing a tight corset when running. She kept on fainting as it was simply too tight. She admitted the corset was to help keep her body in shape, and the medication to help her lose weight. A doctor signed the order.

Protein, creatine, BCAAs (more protein) and **Nitrix** body-building supplements. A sports doctor had prescribed all this for a sixteen-year-old boy. We made the lad take a blood test, and his kidney functions tests were not good. But he never changed his habits. Even after the school banned body-building substitutes, the boys kept on ordering more online, and we cannot keep up, although we try.

Ritalin – some kids on as much as 30–40mg a day. Normally 10mg of quick-acting Ritalin once or twice a day is enough to help a child diagnosed with ADHD concentrate for the duration of the school day. When we questioned the doctor over this large dose, he said the student may not need this every day, but could pick and choose. We refused to do this, and only let him have one day at a time, but he was caught selling it to other students and was 'withdrawn' (read: expelled) from school.

Phenobarbital for migraines. When we researched the other drugs in his tablet, we found it was combined with a benzodiazepine – a highly addictive drug. We were unable to wean him off his daily addiction and I'm sure he's back home with his family, following his doctor's advice, because 'doctor knows best'. No amount of education from any of us, including the school doctor, had an impact. I'm pretty sure the headaches were more a symptom of withdrawal.

Antidepressants and **Ritalin** for depression. The antidepressants might not seem so strange, until I tell you the parents were sending their own by mail because they'd self-diagnosed their child. As for the Ritalin, we never saw a diagnosis of ADHD and there is no medical reason why Ritalin would be prescribed for depression. If he was getting Ritalin when he didn't need it, then he was basically taking hospital quality speed. Speed will make a person feel good for a while, but then they will feel low when it wears off. It could even make any possible depression worse. This is an easy one to deal with – we don't give it.

I could go on for a long time, but I think you see the ethical dilemma we're in. We try to avoid such confusion by informing parents and students that all medicines need a prescription, and that any medication, even over-the-counter medicines, need to go through the health centre. How can I give a medicine, knowing it's wrong, when not only has a doctor prescribed it, but also the parents approve? Legally I can, but I don't. I defer to Dr Fritz who often has a simple solution:

- Make sure the drug is legal for the country we're in. If not, we can't give it.
- If it is legal, but doesn't make sense, request further medical documentation.
- Consider whether the medicine is harmful or harmless – would we cause more harm by stopping its use? In the case of the girl taking thyroxine for no reason, she was devastated when Dr Fritz explained she shouldn't take it, and even after a referral to a specialist she still wouldn't give it up because she just wanted to do what her mum and family doctor said.

Ultimately, as I'm the one dispensing the medicine, I'm the one responsible.

I'm not sure who is to blame for such bizarre treatments; sometimes it's just a case of different places doing medicine differently (which is worrying in itself as we're all made the same), but I suspect the biggest cause is some parents will look for a doctor who will finally give them what they want, no matter what the cost.

Break-a-bone season

Sometimes known as ski season, an average break-a-bone season runs from November to late March and sees:

- two fractured bones a week
- twelve ruined knees, from partial tears to complete ligament ruptures
- one broken back
- one broken neck (fortunately vertebrae only, no spinal damage … yet)
- twenty head injuries, half of whom will end up having a CT scan
- five helicopter evacuations

You may not want to ski after reading such statistics, but it really is a fairly safe sport.

Nine out of ten of the injuries come from jumping. That's why we try to discourage it, but it never works. Even the best get hurt eventually, and Danny was the best of the best.

But he was going to kill himself. Not on purpose, but just as effectively, and maybe even more spectacularly.

'You've got something missing,' I said as I picked out another piece of gravel from his butt cheeks. Danny winced and told me to 'take it easy'.

'What do you mean I've got something missing?'

I'd recently read an article that said that people who have no fear have a physical difference in their brain compared to normal people. It said fearless people have something missing. They were more scientific than 'you've got something missing', but it made a great conversation piece as I relayed this information to Danny – and that's what you want when you're picking stones out of a teenager's bottom, something to distract them.

This wasn't the first time I'd had to patch Danny back together, and I knew it wouldn't be the last, because he took everything to the max. I'd made the naïve mistake of going mountain biking with him and the boys once – never again. He couldn't just enjoy a nice bike ride down the mountain path, through the forest or beside the stream, he had to launch off a ramp and fly as far as he could. He was the most confident mountain biker we had at the school, and landed such jumps nine times out of every ten, but that one time that you miss, that ten per cent guarantee, is when you pay the price. Even with the body armour and helmet, Danny's body kept on getting battered. His latest injury was a graze that began at the ribs and flowed down over his buttock and upper legs, stopping behind the knee, as if a giant tongue of thorns had licked him.

'You don't know fear, it's not normal, it's not healthy. You're going to kill yourself.'

Danny lay grinning at death. 'I know what I'm doing.'

'Jeez, I've never heard a teenager say that before.' My irony was not lost on him.

'Got to die sometime, might as well go doing something you love.'

October

The first snows had left a blanket up high.

The question on everyone's lips was: 'Do you think they'll open early this winter?' At the first sign of snow this is all many of the students can think about and I'm inevitably asked this question multiple times every day. They ask me because I spent eight winters as a ski instructor and ski nurse.

'It's a bit early to say,' I said to Danny and his entourage of dedicated skiers. 'But I wouldn't get too excited if they did open early because the snow won't be that good.' The boys thought my words sacrilege. 'Anytime I can get on the mountain is a good time. There's no such thing as bad snow as long as you can jump,' Danny said, his comment followed by murmurs of agreement.

The boys were referring to the local glacier. I considered an early opening a mixed blessing. While most places started operating their ski-lifts around mid-December, the glacier sometimes opened as early as the first week of November. The glacier itself was pretty flat and provided limited skiing, but it was the jump park that always had me worried. The lads pushed the limits to the max from day one.

I used to tell the students not to jump, which had no effect whatsoever. Instead, I now try to slow them down a bit and tell them to take it easy because they didn't want to ruin their whole season with a break in the first few weeks.

Danny and his friends left my office, promising to take it easy. I wanted to believe them, but I suspected their idea of taking it easy was vastly different from mine.

The first school trip up the mountain was set for first week in November ...

The fifth of November

The news you never want to hear.

SOS, aka ski patrol, had contacted the teacher leading the ski trip to say that Danny had been helicoptered to hospital with serious injuries.

'Serious injuries' could be anything. An image of Danny flying through the air and landing on his head kept replaying in my mind. Was he paralysed? Was he conscious? They don't helicopter people off the mountain for nothing.

It took me forty minutes to drive from school to the hospital.

'Geez mate, the lengths some people go just for a helicopter ride,' I said by way of greeting. Danny was lying in one of the trauma beds, waiting to go to the operating theatre. He raised his head off the bed and wiggled a finger at me as a wave.

'Oh shit man, it's bad,' he said. It looked bad, but I was relieved when I saw him. He was conscious and could move his limbs, well, at least move his legs. The problem was his arms that were both badly broken.

'Pretty sore, eh?'

Danny managed a grin.

'It was pretty bad … but they gave me some good stuff,' he replied, referring to the morphine he'd had in transit.

'Has anyone spoken to your parents yet?' I asked. No one had spoken to them, so it would be up to me to make *the* call.

Danny had crashed going off 'The Monster', the biggest jump in the park. 'I'd already done it three times,' he said, '… it's just bad luck.'

It wasn't bad luck. His one in ten was due, except this time he wasn't going to get away with just gravel in his butt cheeks.

He had fractured both elbows, but his neck, back and skull were fine.

Danny was wheeled to theatre and spent several days in hospital.

The eighth of November

Danny was back in the dorm, and we had a problem.

'I can't reach it,' he said, admitting defeat, a worried frown on his face. 'What am I going to do?'

I thought I'd left this side of nursing behind when I left the hospital, but no nurse ever truly leaves it behind. With his elbows both in plaster, Danny couldn't wipe his butt. I had a hurried conference with my colleagues, none of whom were eager to lend a hand.

'He's going to be in plaster for weeks,' Michaela said. 'We can't go chasing him every time he takes a dump. We physically can't be there.'

She was right, it just wasn't practical … not to mention being deeply embarrassing for Danny. I asked him if he had a preference: 'Do you want me to do it, or one of the girls?'

'You didn't just ask me that, seriously! I don't want anyone wiping my ass, there has to be another way.'

It's humiliating enough having to have someone wipe for you at any stage in life, but as a teenager it must be the worst. Unfortunately, the school simply didn't have the facilities necessary to help Danny out.

'I'm sorry mate, but there is no other way, someone is going to have to do it for you.'

'I just won't wipe it then.' Was he joking?

'*You* didn't just say that!' He managed a chuckle.

'I know you like my butt, sir, but you're not getting that close to it.'

In an ideal world, someone with a serious injury should be sent home, or a parent should come and stay with them. Danny's parents were originally from Colorado where he'd learned to ski, but they were currently in Nigeria and insisted they couldn't look after him properly there. 'There are no hospitals near where we are,' his mother had said when I'd asked her about having Danny at home with her. 'If there are any problems, we won't be able to see a doctor.'

The only solution was to get his mother to come and stay with him.

At first, she explained she couldn't come out because it was hard to get a flight and besides, 'He's in good hands.' But when we told her that she either came out or we'd be sending him home, she agreed to come to her son's assistance.

Danny visibly relaxed when he heard his mum was on her way … well, a part of him didn't relax.

'You're not wiping my ass, I couldn't live with it,' he said defiantly, and held his movements in check until she arrived, thirty hours later. I imagine it was quite the welcome present.

Danny's mum was a pleasant surprise. She really did want to be with her son, but the logistics of being near to care don't always work out when your loved ones are spread over the globe.

'I should have come immediately, I'm sorry,' was a phrase she repeated often, and I can understand the guilt. It's hard to know your child is injured and not be there in a flash. Danny and his mother moved into one of the school apartments, and fortunately the oil company she worked for was very understanding and she was able to stay with him for three weeks, after which he finally regained the use of his elbows.

Danny skied again the following season, although he did stop jumping. He had two permanent reminders not to: a right arm that straightened nearly perfectly, and a left elbow that he was still working on. 'It's pretty good' he often said as he tried to straighten it all the way out and failed. I guess 'pretty good' is good enough to remind him to take life a bit easier.

Caio and Celeste

All mountain schools boast about their ski programme; most make it mandatory, but nothing is really mandatory when you're dealing with someone else's children. Indeed, it's sometimes hard to make anything mandatory when it's your own flesh and blood.

I feel that everyone should ski, and I like the fact the school made it compulsory. But not everyone likes to ski. At first I tried my hardest to encourage the kids, simply because it's a great form of exercise, but after my first winter season at the school, I changed my mind …

0800 hours

Michaela, Justine and I were becoming more frustrated with every letter we read. Today was the first day of skiing for the kids and it was already turning into a nightmare.

We'd spent the last three weeks reminding students and parents that if their child was not able to ski, they must send us a letter with a doctor's certificate. We had very few responses until the day they were due to hit the piste. Out of 400 potential skiers, 100 of them would not be skiing.

'… Caio has an allergy to the cold, and cannot ski …' I showed the letter to Michaela. 'You've got to be kidding,' she said, before handing me another letter from a parent she had received. It was from the mother of Celeste, a good-natured American girl from Florida.

It read: 'Celeste gets sick at altitude and cannot go up the mountain.' It didn't make sense. Celeste's mum was an intelligent woman, a diplomat at the embassy. How could she expect us to believe such rubbish? Celeste already lived at a high altitude – they sent her to a boarding school in the Alps!

'If they don't want to ski, they should just say so. It's embarrassing,' I remarked. Skiing was a luxury I couldn't afford when I was at school, and it felt wrong that a healthy young man or woman should choose not to ski. How could they not like it? Do they even know their parents wrote a letter excusing them? Is it the parents that don't want them to ski, or are the children reluctant to go? I needed to find out first hand what the real story was. I chose Caio's case, and Michaela took up Celeste's. I called Caio into my office.

Like all true Italians, Caio was on the football team and at sixteen years of age, in prime health.

'You live on a mountain. There's snow three months of the year and it gets cold,' I said as I handed him his mother's letter. It wasn't the least confrontational way to start a conversation, but I expected Caio to man-up. Instead, he shrugged his shoulders, and said it's true.

'No one is allergic to the cold, it's not possible,' I said, my tone disbelieving. I was breaking one of the earliest lessons I'd learnt as a junior nurse – never say something is impossible because there are always exceptions, and never box yourself into a corner – but Caio insisted he could not ski, especially today as it was particularly cold.

'I can probably go in the spring, when it's sunny.' He explained that the cold gives him a rash, although he did concede that he

140

might be able to go in the winter months if it was a particularly nice day, but not today, too cold and cloudy.

'So what your mum is really saying, is that you can ski, but only when you want to?' With not the slightest shred of shame, he said that was exactly right.

I stayed calm … because he *was* going to ski.

'Sorry mate, but we need to have an actual medical certificate, signed by a doctor. You're going to have to ski.' Caio sat there quietly, staring at me, his eyes trying to lock onto mine, but I turned to my computer to document the encounter.

'OK, I'll see you later then, and you'll see for yourself.' He left my office and I felt very unsure. His reaction wasn't normal; he didn't call his mother, and he didn't argue. Perhaps you can be allergic to the cold.

Michaela fared no better with Celeste. 'I'm allergic to heights. I get dizzy when I'm at altitude.' Michaela was trying to ascertain if she was sensitive to the altitude, or if she was scared of heights, and asked her if she was worried about going on a chairlift.

'I'm not scared of the chair, it's the altitude, I can't be at altitude.'

'But you're already at altitude, 1600-metres altitude to be exact.' Michaela was doing a better job of staying calm and rational than I had. 'Why would your parents send you here if the altitude makes you sick?'

'This is as high as I can go. Any higher and I get sick.' Michaela reassured her that she wouldn't be going any higher.

'You're a beginner; you'll be at the bottom of the village. It's only 1500 metres, so you'll be fine.' Celeste tried to protest, but she soon realised she'd trapped herself and went to get ready.

There was no way we could see 100 children by lunchtime, when lessons started, so to play it safe, those we couldn't get to see that day were excused, just in case their concerns were legitimate.

1530 hours

Caio walked into the health centre, his face and neck covered in red blotches.

'They're called hives, sir.' He tried sounding sorry, but failed. He couldn't hide the hint of satisfaction in his tone. 'This is your fault.'

It was my fault. Who the hell would have thought that someone could be allergic to the cold? If only I'd listened to him.

He sat with me as I googled 'cold allergy' and found out all I needed to know about 'cold urticaria'.

'... for example, swimming in cold water is the most common cause of a severe, whole-body reaction – leading to fainting, shock and even death ...' The more I read the more relaxed and cheerful Caio became.

Thank goodness I hadn't made him go swimming.

'So, you really can't go out in the cold?' Caio wasn't vindictive, but he did relish his victory, up until the last paragraph, which said he could go out in the cold if he took antihistamines before exposure.

'I don't suppose you thought to take one before going up?' I asked. He shrugged his shoulders and with a mischievous grin said, 'I'm not a nurse.'

Caio's hives resolved with an antihistamine and warmth. He didn't tell his mum, and he did forgive me, while I admitted defeat. From then on, Caio got to pick and choose his ski days.

1615 hours

I found Celeste lying on the examination table in the doctor's office. She'd been taken there by ski patrol after falling and hurting her knee.

'I dislocated my knee,' she said as I walked in. I've never seen a dislocated knee, very few people have. What they usually mean is they've dislocated their patella, or knee-cap, which is far more common. But Celeste seemed happy with either diagnosis, just as long as she didn't have to ski.

The x-ray was normal, and as there was no bruising or swelling, she was discharged with a knee brace, crutches and told not to ski for the next two weeks.

I grabbed her things as she hobbled out the office, and with no hint of guile, asked me, 'Do you think I'll be able to ski again?'

'I hope so, Celeste. I hope so.'

By the time I got Celeste to her dorm, she had ditched the crutches as they were too awkward, and taken off to show her friends her new brace. She also declined the analgesia Dr Fritz had prescribed.

'Mum doesn't like me taking pills,' she added after I suggested that perhaps her knee wasn't as sore as she made out.

Dr Fritz saw her again after her first week with the brace, whereupon he prescribed a two-week course of physiotherapy.

When the physiotherapist couldn't find anything wrong, but the knee still sore, Celeste was eventually sent for an MRI; her parents had insisted. The scan was completely normal, and she finally gave up the brace. But by now she'd missed the first month of lessons, and because her parents did not want their daughter doing such a dangerous sport, she spent ski days sitting in class, surfing the internet on her laptop. Celeste didn't ski for the rest of the season.

Do I think Celeste was faking? Maybe. The difficulty with ski season is that you can't really make someone ski, because it's easy to have a fall and fake an injury, and I see this all the time. But you can never assume they're faking, or lying about an illness, because they'll prove you wrong, as happened with Caio.

143

Unfortunately, the time and effort going into dealing with the repercussions of forcing someone who doesn't want to ski is not sustainable, especially as there are plenty of actual injuries to keep you occupied …

Igor

There are some students you wish had never laid eyes on skis, let alone strap on a pair.

'He went too big,' said some.

'Such sick air,' said others, who had caught the moment on their iPhone.

I'll admit, the image on the phone did look impressive, but 270 degrees is 90 short of a full 360, and the end result is always the same – a nasty landing with a bruise or break. The skier's weight multiplied by speed and gravity meant the energy went from his shoulder and deep into his body.

SOS called me at 4pm informing me they were dropping Igor at the doctor's office. They suspected a fractured clavicle, or collarbone, and felt the quickest and most effective treatment could be received here in the village.

'It needs surgery,' declared Igor. He was quickly told to be quiet by the doctor. Dr Fritz could put up with long hours, midnight call-outs, indecent referrals (i.e., unnecessary referrals to specialists), a round at the local hospital *and* an average eighty-hour work week, but he could not tolerate disrespect, especially

145

from rude, loud and demanding teenagers.

'He can't tell me to shut up,' Igor said, turning his attention to me for support.

'If I were you, I'd shut up,' I recommended.

Before he could voice a protest he cried out in pain.

'Fuck, fuck, fuck … what the fuck are you doing? Find someone who knows what they're doing. Take me to a real hospital.' Dr Fritz was trying to remove Igor's jacket so he could send him to have an x-ray, but he wasn't going to argue with Igor.

Dr Fritz's waiting room looked sick. It was overflowing with people in various states of ski dress, clutching arms, legs resting on chairs, bandages pressed against bleeding foreheads, and even holding bowls ready to empty their stomach contents into. It was crowded, noisy, and the height of the winter ski season. Dr Fritz saw no reason to treat someone who didn't want his care.

'Goodbye then,' he said and left the room. Dr Fritz has always been a man of few words, and it seems to work. Igor was so surprised he briefly forgot his pain.

'He can't walk out, he has to see me.' With my patience drained, I turned to Igor.

'I know you're sore, but if you don't show some manners, you'll be taking a taxi to hospital.' Igor wasn't listening, his fingers were flying over his iPhone. I added: 'If I were you, I'd say sorry,' but he took no heed.

'It's for you,' Igor declared, holding his phone out to me. I made no move to grab it as I knew what it would be: an angry parent or an agent. I can't decide who's worse, angry parents in broken English, or fluent agents paid to put me in my place.

As if I'd wondered aloud, Igor added: 'It's my agent, he wants to talk to you.' I took a deep breath, and tried to relax before grabbing the phone.

'Is this the doctor?'

I told the man on the phone that I was the nurse.

'You have to take Igor to hospital now. We do not want a ...' He paused as he searched for the right word. 'We do not want a simple village doctor to treat Igor.' The way he stressed the word 'simple' was not an accident that comes from speaking a foreign language.

It was time to take control.

'Excuse me, but who am I talking to, and what relation are you to Igor?' A reasonable request spoken in a reasonably firm tone got a reasonable response.

'I'm Victor and I am speaking on behalf of the family.'

Victor could be anybody, an agent sitting in an office in Moscow, representing many families, or someone working solely for Igor's family. His whole life could be Igor and his clan.

Sometimes we never have any direct contact with a blood relative, even in very serious instances – some of our children have trouble even getting hold of their mother or father. It's not always easy knowing who to call. For all I know, Igor (if that's even his real name) could be the son of a powerful politician or criminal mob boss, although some people might say they're one and the same.

'Igor must be taken to hospital now,' the voice on the end of the line told me. 'I kindly ask you to do as the family request.'

I could put Igor in the car and take him to hospital, but that would be the wrong thing to do. He'd suffer while I drove down the winding mountain road, the combination of pain and such movement would probably cause him to vomit, and he'd get no better treatment. I tried to explain this to Victor and Igor.

'Dr Fritz sees these sorts of injuries all the time. I have complete faith in him.'

'I don't care if you have full confidence. You're not a doctor, and we want an expert. You will do something now.'

These sorts of characters should only exist in fiction, a Bond film, but I've learned they are real.

When I explained that the hospital would be busy because it was the weekend and Igor would have to wait hours, in pain, before even being seen, Victor simply requested we go to an even bigger hospital. 'Igor's father has ordered you to do this.'

I don't mind being told what to do, having worked in fast-paced medical teams you get used to it, but I don't carry out orders that will ultimately cause more suffering for my patient, even an unpleasant patient. I ended the conversation and turned my attention back to Igor.

Dr Fritz came back to see Igor, and the x-ray confirmed a fractured right collarbone, but he was lucky because it was a simple break, in the middle of the bone and while the ends weren't in complete alignment, they weren't too badly displaced. I've seen much worse.

If you took a stick of celery and bent until it snapped, and then slid each end of the break up a few millimetres, it would look a bit like Igor's x-ray.

Igor continued his tirade.

'I'm not wearing a shitty brace.' He was objecting to the standard treatment (at least in some parts of the world) of a soft brace that pulls the shoulders back.

'Fine,' replied Dr Fritz, placing the brace back in the cupboard. He handed Igor some painkillers, placed his arm in a simple sling, and told him to leave the office.

With breaks like Igor's, casts are out of the question. The brace wasn't even absolutely necessary, and some doctors never use it, but the theory is that by pulling the shoulders back, you help pull the fracture back into line. Sometimes it helps, sometimes not, but either way the bone heals by itself with rest.

'You can't throw me out!' Igor demanded.

But Igor's treatment was finished.

I took Igor back to his dorm and settled him in for the night.

Part two

It came as no surprise when Igor went to see a specialist orthopaedic surgeon. His parents would have it no other way, and Dr Fritz was happy to pass him on. Unfortunately I was there when the surgeon told Igor the good news.

'You don't need surgery.' Igor couldn't hide his disappointment and resorted to what all fourteen-year-old children say when they're at a loss. 'But Mum said I need surgery.' The surgeon shook his head. 'There's no benefit. It will heal fine. Surgery is not only unnecessary, but risky.' He added that when you operate in such an area there can be problems with healing, as well as the risk of causing damage to the surrounding tissue.

'There's a lot of nerves and blood vessels that could be damaged,' he pointed to a model of a shoulder on his desk to illustrate his point. 'In this case, surgery would be the wrong thing to do.'

Igor's parents were unsatisfied because it was our village doctor who had made the referral, and they wanted an opinion from an orthopaedist that they had found themselves. Victor re-emerged, in real life this time, and took Igor to the specialist the family had found. They were told exactly the same thing.

I never got to exchange pleasantries with Victor and only managed to see the outline of a hulking frame dressed in a black suit with matching sunglasses, dwarfing the driver's seat of a Mercedes, cigarette hanging from lower lip. He was more real and sinister than any film.

It's good that some people have the chance to shop around for second, or even third, opinions, but it's a bit pointless shopping around when you don't listen. If you've got enough money, you'll eventually find someone to voice the opinion you want. I see this sort of thing a lot, and it can be dangerous. I used to think it was about culture, East versus West, but it's a culture that transcends nations – the culture of money.

Three doctors' opinions in two weeks was not enough and we were told Igor was going to be flown home.

'I'm going home for an operation.' Igor still sounded angry, but it wasn't directed at us, it was at the whole health system of this country. 'We have proper doctors in Russia. They'll know what to do.' I couldn't believe any doctor would be crazy enough to operate on him given that two top orthopaedic doctors, from a country famed for its skiing and fractures, had said 'no'.

Igor returned four weeks later with the scar to show where the metalwork had gone in.

As far as medical treatment goes, anything is possible when you've got enough money, but it doesn't always equate with better care. In a world where medicine is big business, it's getting harder and harder for nurses – who work every day on the frontline – to be heard.

The staff

It's not just the students I look after. Sometimes I'm a nurse for the big kids as well.

I don't think the average person really knows what a nurse does although that didn't stop my friends asking how many 'butts' I'd wiped during my college days, and I always responded by saying I'd give them all their medication rectally, if they were ever admitted. Fortunately, the teachers I work alongside don't ask such crude questions, but they still have a very limited understanding of what I do.

'See the nurse' they say for the most minor cut or runny nose. They say it because I'm their resident medical expert, always happy to see anyone, whether it is a student or faculty member.

I've treated Mr Huang, the PE teacher, who had foot warts and had heard that I had some cryogenic therapy in a can, which I did. I offered him one course of treatment, but insisted he see the doctor for follow-up.

Mr Sapsford, a science teacher, for a rash around his groin, upper thighs and buttocks. An intense deep red, that was itchy. I referred him to the doctor who had no idea what it was, and it took a dermatologist to diagnose scabies. I'd seen scabies a number of times, but never like this.

Miss Crowther, the library assistant had nits. Her dorm had been battling recurring outbreaks of head lice all term. I didn't have the heart to tell her that her infestation was so thick she was likely the source of the ongoing problem, although she probably got the hint when I said I'd rarely seen them so abundant.

Miss Hunter, an English teacher, wanted to know if I could give her one of our 'emergency' contraceptives, commonly known as the morning after pill. I sent her to the pharmacy. She was relieved when I explained you can get it over the counter.

At the school we have 100 teachers and dorm parents, alongside another 100 support staff from builders, cooks, cleaners, receptionists, gardeners and more, and while the official policy is that I'm not responsible for them and do not have to treat them, I can't exactly say no. It's hard to turn them away, but sometimes when you cross the line between a friend and a nurse things can get … awkward, as I discovered when I met Claire at a staff game of touch rugby.

Claire was sporty. She had shapely calves, toned thighs, and could bike faster and run longer than anyone else at school. She was also cute; even as a happily-married family man, I could see that. Understandably she was popular and the only reason we were playing touch was because of Claire, and because she was also from New Zealand.

'Too slow,' she called as she side-stepped my clumsy attempt to stop her, and scored her third try. She was not only fast, but like all kiwis, rugby was a large part or her DNA.

'Did you play much?' she asked as she threw the ball in my direction. I'm pretty sure every kiwi has played rugby at some stage, even if only once. 'Yeah, a bit,' I replied. Such a lie! Thankfully, whilst I may be the only Kiwi missing the 'league' gene, none of the staff – 95 per cent of whom are from America and Britain – needed to know that.

By the time the game had finished, Claire was the only one showing no signs of suffering. But that's because she was only 25 – at least a decade younger than most of us. At the end of the game, there were some tweaked knees, limping ankles, grazed skin and bruised egos – nothing too serious – but they all asked me for my opinion.

I told them to wait and see. 'It's too early to tell, but you're still walking, so it'll probably be fine.' And it usually is. A bit of reassurance is all most people need.

Then, a few days later, Claire hobbled into my office.

'I fell off my bike,' she said by way of a greeting, and began to take down her jeans.

'Hold on … slow down a bit,' I stammered. 'Why don't you tell me what's wrong first?'

'I'm sure you've seen it all before,' she declared, immune to my protests. 'It's pretty badly bruised. I just want to know if there is anything you can do.' What I could do is get Michaela to have a look, but she told me not to bother. 'Just look at my hip, that's all.'

Her skin was a ripe black and blue, extending from the crest of the right hip, all the way down the side of her leg, ending midway down her thigh. 'What the hell were you doing? That's some fall you've had.' It would take weeks to heal completely, but she said it wasn't a particularly big fall. 'I wasn't jumping … just landed awkwardly.' I recommended she get an x-ray, but she was reluctant to go. 'Can't you just give me some cream or something?' I explained I was worried that she might have a small chip broken off her hip, or something more. 'I want you to check your urine, to make sure there's no blood in it.'

Despite my advice, she was still reluctant to see Dr Fritz. In the end, I took her to see him myself.

An x-ray showed Claire had chipped her hip bone, although her urine was clear. Treatment involved regular ibuprofen and gel to apply topically (which means, on the surface).

'Thanks for everything – I didn't think it was so bad. I owe you one.'

But, Claire never did pay me back. Especially not after 'the incident' ...

Two months later

Claire had just returned from the Christmas break. Nearly everyone heads away for the break, the British to Britain, the Americans to somewhere warmer, with a beach and palm trees, and the Kiwis to wherever their hearts desire. I spent Christmas at school with family.

The night before school was about to start up again, I received a message on my phone.

'Can I see you soon? Urgent. Claire.'

I called her straight back and she said she was in terrible pain, and I agreed to see her in the health centre.

Claire couldn't sit still. 'It hurts so much, I don't know what to do.' I asked her what was wrong, and she became shy, reluctant to share. 'It's so embarrassing, but it's so sore, you have to help me.'

I promised I wouldn't tell a soul, and suggested that she didn't have to tell me; that I could take her to hospital, but she knew what was wrong.

'I can't poo.'

A chuckle escaped.

'It's not funny,' she snapped. 'It's so sore.'

I asked how long since she last had one.

'Two weeks, I haven't had a poo in two weeks.'

'Shit.'

'Yes, shit,' she echoed.

I asked her what she'd tried so far to fix the problem. She said she'd tried liquids, tablets, and even suppositories. 'And they didn't help, even a little?'

She shook her head. 'It's just there, like concrete. I feel like I'm trying to pass a brick.'

'You really need to go to hospital, I'll drive you there.'

But she refused to go. 'Can't you do something, like, you know ...'

I did know something that would work, but it didn't feel right, so I asked Claire if she would mind if I called Michaela for some backup.

'I don't care who you get, as long as they can help.'

I have no problem with getting down and dirty, but Claire was a colleague, a friend, and, most importantly, a woman.

We did have an enema in stock, but I handed the problem over to Michaela.

I don't think you need much more detail. Suffice to say, the enema Claire received was not quite enough, and Michaela said she had to give a little, er, encouragement, but the problem was fixed, and Claire was eternally grateful. But there has been no offer to pay me back because she 'owed' me one. In fact, she has avoided Michaela and me ever since.

Foodies

It's not just the teachers that require some medical advice. It's the maintenance, domestic and kitchen staff too. And you can forget about office hours; they approach me anytime, about anything … a lot.

I first met Raj during breakfast.

'Can you please be giving me something for my stomach?' Raj asked as he charged into my office, hopping from one foot to the next, as if barely able to contain himself.

I'd only ever seen glimpses of Raj in the kitchen or serving up meals in the cafeteria. I'd never spoken with him before, but he looked in pain.

'What's wrong?' I replied. 'Perhaps you should be at home.'

'No, no, no. I'll be fine, I just need something to stop the diarrhoea.' I normally don't give anything for diarrhoea, at least in the first 24 hours of a bug, as it's a normal part of the illness. Instead, I encouraged him to drink and told him that the diarrhoea should settle down on its own in a day or two.

'But it's been three days already.'

I paused, and kept the forkful of scrambled egg I was about to ingest, in mid-air.

'But you're at work?'

Raj started at me blankly; he seemed to be trying to figure out what I was trying to say.

'It's OK,' he finally said. 'I'm not asking for any time off, I'll be fine.' I placed my fork and egg back down on the plate.

If someone has diarrhoea for three days, I'd normally refer him or her to the doctor, at least if it was serious and frequent, which Raj explained his was.

'It's exploding very much,' he said, almost cheerfully, when I asked how bad it was. That would explain the hopping on his feet. He really was trying to hold it in.

I referred him to the doctor, and told him he couldn't work in the kitchen.

'No doctor. It's OK.' He waved his arms, brushing off my suggestions, before leaving me to eat my breakfast in peace.

I forgot about Raj, until later that day …

Raj seemed a bit better – he was no longer hopping.

He served up lunch, a curry, a brown curry, to me as well as every student who walked into the cafeteria.

For some reason, I couldn't eat the curry; it looked too loose, and besides, I don't eat enough fruit anyway. I made do with an apple and banana.

The next morning twenty cases of gastroenteritis were reported.

I was suddenly very grateful I'd taken the healthy option the previous lunch. Something had to be done. As soon as all twenty cases had been dealt with, I entered the bowels of the kitchen.

There were a dozen kitchen staff in total, including Raj, all curious, all unaware.

'I just want to find out what your policy is in the case of illness,' I asked delicately, fearing a backlash. Instead, they stared at each other for answers, before shrugging their shoulders and grinning.

'What happens if you have diarrhoea?' Again, I drew a blank.

'You do know you need to be diarrhoea free for at least 48 hours before working in a kitchen.' I finally got a response. They all began laughing.

'What's so funny?' I asked, and Raj spoke up.

'If we did that, no one would ever be at work.' The conversation was over as they dispersed to their various stations to prepare the next meal.

I don't eat at school anymore. And neither do half the students.

I wrote a letter to the headmaster outlining my concerns, and I was told that they'd looked into it. But I never heard from anyone about it again.

Since the scene in the kitchen, Raj stopped coming to me when he was sick. In fact, I've not seen anyone from the food crew in the health centre in many years.

We still do get regular outbreaks of diarrhoea and vomiting, it just never goes away. And from the discussions I've had with other school nurses at various conferences, the matter of food quality and food hygiene at schools can be hit or miss; some schools have great food, some mediocre, some disturbing. We seem to be somewhere in the middle. While the occasional mass-event stomach upset is wrong – especially if you know the root cause – I have learned that the best school nurses have to choose their battles wisely. Especially when you're dealing with the boss ...

Priorities

Dear Mr Driscoll,

After our recent boarding school conference, we discovered we
were the only school out of 60 that does not have defibrillators.
Can we please remedy this?'

Sincerely,
   The health centre

Attendees at a conference I had recently been to were shocked
– not literally, thank goodness – that we didn't have any defibrillators on campus, and horrified when I explained how isolated
we were.

I don't usually like being the centre of a confrontation, but after
my letter, Mr Driscoll called a meeting with the nurses.

'In all your years here, have we ever needed one?' Mr Driscoll
asked. I reminded him that Dr Fritz had used one during a cross-
country running event, but as Dr Fritz was actually in attendance
during the event, we hadn't needed one of our own.

'But kids don't have heart attacks.'

He was right, they don't really have heart attacks in the traditional sense, where a clot blocks an artery, the patient just suddenly collapses and their heart goes into life threatening rhythms.

'But it's not just the kids, there's over 100 staff here.' I kept my cool, because surely he'd see that the one-off cost of 5000 euros for three defibrillators spread throughout campus was worth every penny. 'And have you seen how many of your workers smoke and drink, and how old they are?'

Mr Driscoll was unfazed, so I pulled out the big guns.

'Take Mr Rodgers, for example.' I was referring to our beloved art teacher, due to retire at the end of the year. 'He's just had a heart attack.' It's helpful that the weekend the medical staff were away at the conference that inspired my plea, learning about our deficiencies, Mr Rodgers had a heart attack.

Mr Driscoll didn't answer straight away, perhaps because there was no answer to this, but he came up with something.

'He's OK, he's going to be fine. He wasn't shocked. The emergency services were fantastic.'

Mr Rodgers was down the mountain in the city when he'd turned grey and clutched his chest in pain. His wife had taken him to the emergency room where they treated him with clot busting drugs, and saved his heart from being damaged. He hadn't needed a defibrillator, but that was because of his rapid treatment. Any longer, and he probably would have.

'Listen, this conference you went to was run by Americans, right?' I could read his mind, but I nodded my head and kept silent.

'We all know they overdo things.'

'Do you not care about your staff?' I dared, and Mr Driscoll took the bait.

'You're walking a fine line.'

It seems I'm always walking a fine line, but why is doing the right thing such a risky business? Whether it's working in a hospital or a school, the battle is the same. Management want to save money, staff just want to do what's right.

'So, we're not going to get any?' Mr Driscoll was fuming. Instead of answering he shook his head and stormed out.

'Can I get that in writing?' I said to his retreating back, but he didn't pause, and I never got an official written reply.

I had to get creative.

I asked the people in charge of raising donations for the school to ask families if they could donate money to the good cause, but they said no.

'It doesn't look good asking money for something we should already have.'

'It would look a lot worse if someone keels over and dies when we could have saved them,' I retaliated.

I began a campaign of annoyance, and regularly bombarded management with written requests for defibrillators, which generally went like this:

'I hope you don't mind me putting it in writing, but I can't accept responsibility if one of the students or staff dies because we don't have a defibrillator. The decision and responsibility is yours.'

I knew that when you put requests like this in writing, they *have* to reply. I learnt that from my time working in hospitals. In fact, in hospitals, if you didn't put it in writing, you didn't do it. It's one of the reasons so many nurses are compelled to spend more time in the office than with their patients.

Shockingly, management didn't reply; yet another reminder I was no longer an A&E nurse.

It took four years, but finally we got them. Our sheer tenacity paid off. All the nurses brought up the issue of defibrillators every chance we got, either at a staff meeting, or further written requests.

We even sourced out the best deals and managed to include a training course for the whole faculty as part of the package. Financially, it was now more attractive as it wasn't just 5000 euros for the health centre, but 5000 euros to cover compulsory training for all the staff. It's a shame that it took so long, but, for the sake of the children and the staff, I'm proud that I kept on fighting for them. We haven't used them yet … but it's nice to know that they're there.

Payback

I didn't really know what to say, and that in itself is saying a lot because I am rarely left tongue tied, but the headmaster was deadly serious. 'Is there any risk of infection?' he asked again, while I busily searched for an answer on Google.

Meanwhile, Adam sat on the edge of the examination table unsure how to react. I think he was trying to look upset, worried, angry and disgusted all at the same time. I just hoped my face was not as transparent as his because I was having difficulty keeping it straight.

Adam and Bryce had enrolled halfway through the first term and had found themselves roommates. It takes time to adjust to a new school, particularly in your senior year and especially when joining mid-term as there are questions which are rarely left unasked, such as: why anyone would transfer in their senior year? Did they get kicked out from their last school? Are they troublemakers? Was it drugs? Even if the reason is benign, the speculation is usually not. The school gives these students a chance, an officially clean slate, but we sit, we wait and we wonder.

When two seventeen-year-old boys are thrust together in a new environment they're never themselves; they're two egos trying to appear strong, desperate to fit in and become popular. By mid-term the social groups are already well established and newcomers sometimes struggle. To fit in they do silly things, all for a laugh, and what's better than laughing at someone else's expense? Sadly not all teenagers know when to say enough is enough.

It began one evening when Bryce was absent and Adam herded half a dozen lads into his room – 'bring your phones guys, this is going online' – and proceeded to play his prank.

The following evening Bryce was confused and angered by the behaviour of the other boys in the dorm. No one would sit near him, some started calling him 'shithead' or 'shit for brains'; he had no idea why until a message arrived in his inbox. Bryce clicked on the link and watched a video of Adam as he picked up Bryce's pillow and farted loudly into it.

How should he react? How would you react? In the old days (time before the internet) it wouldn't be such a big deal because you might have heard that someone's buttocks had been intimate with your pillow, but now you not only saw it in high definition, the rest of the school did too, making retaliation compulsory, and it would need to be equally as public.

'He's going to fucking pay!' Bryce shouted. The boys, iPhones at the ready, followed Bryce as he made his way from the study hall in search of Adam. But such a crowd couldn't pass through the dorm unnoticed and probably saved Adam from a certain brawl, the staff on duty were quick to intervene.

The IT department discovered the video and were eventually able to delete from the school's system, although I'm sure it's still floating somewhere in cyberspace, no doubt forever.

Adam received a full weekend of detention, a small price to pay for the prestige he earned. In the minds of every student on campus justice had not been served.

Thankfully, once the heat of the moment had passed, the boys chose to be men and made an effort to get along. No one said 'I'm sorry' or 'I forgive you', that's not how young men talk to each other. Instead, they played at fighting, shared links to some online porn (determined students always find ways around firewalls) and even backed each other when empty beer cans were found in the room.

Then, one morning about two weeks after the pillow incident, or 'butt-gate' as it became known, Adam woke and felt something not quite right with his eyes, and when he looked in the mirror he saw that both of his eyes were red and watery.

'Is it pink-eye?' he asked and I said that it certainly looked that way. Pink-eye is the expression Americans use for conjunctivitis. If it looks mild, and there is no discharge (crust or pus), then the modern treatment is to wait for a day or two as it often resolves on its own. In this instance, because there had been pus I chose not to wait to see the doctor.

With a simple course of antibiotics his eyes should have got better, but after three days they had become worse and so his treatment was upped.

That same week, another video surfaced amongst the students and this time it featured Bryce pulling down his pants and very liberally 'smearing' his bare arse on Adam's pillow. Butt-gate had escalated to 'smear-gate'.

I'd never heard of anyone contracting conjunctivitis through a pillow that had been in contact with someone's buttocks, but apparently it is not unheard of. I'm sure Bryce had no idea such a thing could happen, and hadn't wanted Adam to get ill. Either way, it didn't matter if he knew or not because revenge had not only been served, but served in a very public way. For weeks after, Adam was continually asked if he had been 'poo-faced'.

Some students thought Bryce had 'crossed a line' because bare buttocks were involved – others thought it genius. Regardless, everyone felt Adam had been 'owned' and the score settled.

None of the faculty would have found out about the latest video had it not been for a careless slip of the tongue. There's always one student who can't keep their mouth shut and 'accidentally' says too much to a teacher, and that was how Mr Driscoll became involved. But it was to no avail. Adam and Bryce kept their traps shut and denied any such feud, while Adam's eyes continued to weep. It took a visit to an ophthalmologist and a third course of medication to clear it.

Surprisingly, the boys claimed they didn't hate each other throughout any of this. Bryce even said as much to me, with a shrug: 'It just got a bit out of hand.' One thing is for sure … this wasn't the last time a bit of fun went bad …

When the fun goes bad

Part one

Most of the pranks I witness at school are harmless. Even Bryce and Adam's brief feud didn't cause any real damage. But you can never tell what will happen when boys will be boys …

It began with a sausage. Not a banger or hotdog – a twelve-inch-thick, meaty sausage. The sausage that started the whole mess belonged to Pablo.

'Come and try zee sore-sage. Vee know vous want ze taste.' There are some things that most guys will always laugh at; farting, and walking around with a sausage hanging out your trousers. I shouldn't join in the laughter at Pablo's antics, but in a school full of kids, I'm still the biggest kid I know.

'Give it a rest, Pablo. I'm sure you've got some homework to do,' I said, trying to be the mature grown-up. 'We've had some fun, but it's study hall and I've got patients to see.'

Pablo returned to his room, sausage safely tucked away. I headed towards Room 45 to see Max, a boy who had been complaining of stomach cramps and nausea. It's always helpful to see someone looking miserable, not because I like to see people suffer, but because it brings out my better side. It brings out the nurse in me;

the parent in me. Max was curled up in a ball on his bed, hands clutching his mid-section, and his face pale.

Medicine is rarely exact and it took me ten minutes to diagnose a probable viral gastroenteritis. He had no fever and no signs of appendicitis (although that could change at any time), and the onset of diarrhoea was oddly reassuring. Max would be OK with rest. Mere moments after I left his room I heard a blood-curdling scream echoing down the corridor. I ran towards it.

Pablo was kneeling on the hallway floor, clutching his face, blood steadily seeping through his fingers. His shirt was already soaked. Standing over him, armed with a broom handle, was Azamat. At sixteen years of age, Azamat was small by Kazak standards, but even small guys can be pushed too far.

'So … so … so … sorry … so sorry,' Azamat squeaked. The makeshift weapon fell from his fingers. 'I didn't mean to.' Two teachers had arrived. I asked one to take Azamat away and the other to keep the rest of the kids in their rooms.

Pablo was a head taller than Azamat, but like David slaying Goliath, it looked like the smaller man had broken Pablo's nose with one hit. A bloody, broken nose will nearly always knock your opponent down.

I took Pablo straight to Dr Fritz while Pablo was being x-rayed to confirm the break, I was able to ascertain the full story.

Pablo had been playing with his sausage again and chased Azamat down the corridor with it hanging out of his trousers. Azamat had told him to 'fuck off', but Pablo had not let up. He caught Azamat off-guard as he pretended to ram him from behind and had told him to 'bend over, and take ze sausage like a good little boy!' whereupon Azamat snapped and lashed out.

Rarely is an assault a simple matter. It would always be much easier if there were a designated asshole who deserved it, but Pablo wasn't a bad guy. He was just a kid who took a prank too far with the wrong person. That seems to be the way most problems get out of hand.

Azamat felt awful.

'I didn't mean to. I'm sorry. It's all my fault ...' Azamat had retreated to his room. When I returned I found him sitting cross-legged on his couch, rocking back and forth. 'It's my fault, all my fault.'

He not only accepted full responsibility, he didn't even try to defend his actions. There was no 'he started it' or 'he made me angry'.

Naturally, this matter was a huge deal, but after many discussions both families agreed that Azamat could stay at the school on the condition that he have anger management counselling.

I was pleased that he would be staying because we all make mistakes. The most important thing is to learn from them, and Azamat was genuinely remorseful and willing to learn to deal with his anger, although it was a calculated gamble, because anything can happen when you can't control your anger.

Part two

Even before the sausage incident, Azamat had been the sort of boy who kept to himself. He wasn't a loner, he just liked staying inside.

When others went biking or played sport, he could be found sitting at his desk in symbiosis with his computer. When he needed a break, he migrated to his couch and fired up the Xbox, his eyes glued to the 36-inch flat screen he'd brought with him.

Most of his social interaction at school happened when others came and joined him on the couch, or when someone had a problem only he had the skills to fix.

Everyone knew him as the 'quiet' guy who was good at gaming.

Only a handful of people noticed as he quietly disappeared off everyone's radar altogether.

'He hasn't played in two weeks,' said Yang, Azamat's roommate.

Alongside Cathy the counsellor, the dorm staff and nurses, Yang was keeping an unofficial eye on his roommate. Yang was as addicted to the virtual world as Azamat, and they usually played together in team events or solo, where they'd hunt each other down.

I made a note to tell Cathy this latest piece of news. She was already seeing him two times a week, but every bit of information always helped.

Another week passed and things seemed a bit better. A group of boys had spent Friday night playing with Azamat on his Xbox and Yang even said that things seemed more normal.

'He seemed pretty happy,' Yang said, referring to Friday night. 'It's been a long time since I saw him like that.'

Cathy's sessions with Azamat were going well. 'He's starting to open up,' she said, 'although he does feel a lot of shame.' Some shame seems natural, even healthy, but in some cultures shame is more powerful or harmful than others. I asked Cathy if he'd said anything about his family, and she shook her head.

'We haven't got that far yet, and his parents haven't responded to my emails.' It's often hard dealing with some parents, especially when they come from backgrounds like Azamat's. Often Kazak families are traditional, patriarchal, as in the man is the head of the household, and he needs to look and be strong. Children must show respect for their elders, and must avoid bringing dishonour to the family. Family is everything in Kazak society.

'Did he give you any idea how angry they are, or if he was punished?' Not every family treats their child the same when problems arise, and some punishments that are illegal here, are normal elsewhere. Again Cathy admitted to drawing a blank.

One month later I received the most disturbing phone call I've had yet.

At 8.15 on Saturday night Azamat tried to kill himself.

Yang had left the room he shared with Azamat to go into town but before leaving the building he had realised he'd forgotten his wallet and returned a few minutes later to find Azamat with an open bottle of pills and a bottle of vodka. He had seen the bottle before, sitting harmlessly on the desk, a bottle of ibuprofen which he thought had been at least half full.

'If I hadn't forgotten my wallet, he'd be dead.' Yang would need serious help to get over this experience; he would go on to spend a lot of time with Cathy. There was at least one dorm parent who would require counselling as well.

After the incident, Cathy kept berating herself. 'I should have known. I could have done something.'

Fortunately, Azamat had no lasting physical damage from his suicide attempt, and his parents came and took him home. I never heard from Azamat again. No one did.

Any suicide attempt is awful, but there's something especially chilling about teenage suicide. In my ten years as a school nurse, I've seen four other 'attempts', although Azamat's was by far the most serious. The others have been cries for help, students who had overdosed on a handful of paracetamol (because they thought it harmless) then called the nurse. This is not including those who self-harm, of which, sadly, there are too many to mention in this book. Since Azamat's suicide attempt, I've often found myself lying in bed at night mulling over what drives a young person, with the whole world in front of them, to take their life. As a school nurse, and when you experience these types of situations so close up, so *real*, you spend too many nights awake. It's part of the job.

CHAPTER FOUR

The Internet

Swine flu

Part one

It all began over Christmas break. Reports about and the subsequent panic over the swine flu outbreak started to take hold.

'Thank goodness it's in Mexico,' Justine remarked as we sat watching the evening news, but any sense of relief evaporated when I reminded her that we had twenty Mexican students returning to school after the break. 'Oh shit, what are we going to do?'

'Maybe their parents will keep them at home, keep them isolated,' I suggested. It sounded a reasonable and sensible suggestion.

Even if there were no students returning from that part of the world, these things invariably spread. Everyone gets ill to some degree or another over the winter, and with 400 children, plus nearly 100 adults living, working and breathing the same moist, stagnant dorm air, it was only a matter of time before swine flu panic reared its porcine head.

What were we going to do? Firstly, I wasn't going to tell Justine about the horrific YouTube clip I had just watched, and the next thing was to stay calm.

'Half of those infected are dying!' Justine wasn't doing the best job of staying calm. 'Healthy young people are dropping all over the place.' She had determined that the school needed to close and began warning the rest of the faculty just how fatal this new virus was.

As a result, no one was willing to look after anyone with swine flu, and that was before the students even came back from the holidays.

'You're the nurse, it's your job to look after them,' explained Mr Green, the head of the social studies department. He was a methodical, concise speaker who managed to sound reasonable no matter how unreasonable his request, and as such was the natural spokesman for the rest of the faculty. 'I don't get paid enough for this sort of stuff, and neither do any of the staff here. We're not having anything to do with swine flu.'

I don't get paid enough for this sort of stress either, but I wasn't worried about myself getting sick. I was worried about my family getting sick. I'm terrified of bringing home a bug and infecting them.

If there was a major outbreak, there was no way three nurses could handle it. I tried reassuring the staff that they were over-reacting and that the most likely thing to happen would be a few extra cases of flu.

'But you don't know for sure.' I was becoming irritated because Mr Green wanted definite answers, when there weren't even any confirmed cases in Europe yet.

I'd had enough. 'You're right, I don't know for sure. For all we know, everyone could die.' Oddly, he didn't feel reassured.

About the same time the students were returning from break, the first cases of swine flu outside of Mexico were confirmed.

Justine wondered if any of the Mexican students would be coming back. Indeed, they all returned, plus some more. Twenty Mexican students had gone away for break, and twenty-two Mexican students had come back. Two students had been enrolled over the holidays because their parents wanted their children as far from the centre of the outbreak as possible. With such logic, it was no wonder that swine flu became a worldwide event.

Meanwhile, the scare-mongering was only getting worse, not just amongst the faculty, but the students ...

Part two

I couldn't tell if the boys were serious, or just pulling a fast one on me.

'There's a video on YouTube. You have to see it,' Ryan, the loudest of the group, was insisting. I refused to look at any video claiming that vaccinations, especially flu vaccines, were not just potentially harmful, but fatal.

'You can't believe anything you see online,' I protested. 'Do some real research and find out the facts.' Such fighting talk got the reaction it deserved.

'You're not injecting me with poison,' insisted Ryan; the rest were in absolute agreement. There was no way they were going to get the swine flu vaccination, even if their parents insisted. 'You can't make me take it. I know my rights.'

No one can force anyone to take a vaccination, but we'd been in daily contact with Dr Fritz for guidance on how to deal with the problem, and he was getting his recommendations from the health authorities. Because of the school environment, we were instructed to vaccinate everyone, both low and high risk, although we'd need parental consent.

After reassuring the students that no one would be forced to do anything – and that no one should believe what they read on the internet – I did my own 'in-depth' research, and asked Google. I couldn't get a straight answer. The news filtering through was that swine flu wasn't particularly serious for healthy people, but to the old, young, frail and those with chronic diseases, it was deadly.

When the vaccine finally arrived at school, a record 90 per cent of parents requested their child be vaccinated, but only half of the students wanted it.

'You didn't watch the video, did you?' accused Ryan. 'You wouldn't be making us do this if you had.'

We had set up a vaccination booth in the boys' dorm, and things weren't going well. Ryan had become the unofficial anti-vaccine spokesman, and he had made life difficult because he'd posted a link of the YouTube video on Facebook and to the whole school, via the online student conference. I finally agreed to look at the damned thing.

How can something be convincing and unbelievable at the same time? I wished I hadn't looked at the clip, but at least I knew what we were up against. 'She can only walk backwards.' Ryan was kindly acting as narrator for me. 'She had the vaccine, and now she's a freak.'

The clip portrayed a healthy young woman's reaction to a flu vaccine and how it had destroyed her life. She could no longer walk in a straight line, and couldn't speak properly either. The news reporter said the scientists thought she had a rare form of dystonia. It had to be a lie, or a one-in-a-million freak reaction, but it didn't matter because the damage was done.

Ryan didn't get a swine flu shot, or any other shot for that matter. In fact, only half the students finally got the vaccine; it didn't matter that there was no objective data, or that the government health authorities had given their approval for it as well as guidelines for coping with any confirmed cases.

That winter saw no deaths at the school, although we did see a slightly higher number of coughs, colds and fever. Thankfully no one began walking backwards.

We did get one confirmed case – Ryan. He suffered from asthma, and regularly used his inhalers, especially when he had a cold, and as an 'at-risk' patient, the health guidelines insisted he be tested. After an unpleasant few days, he made a full recovery.

How did Ryan catch the virus? We had no idea, but there were probably plenty of others that got swine flu. In fact, there were more cases of flu than normal, but they weren't tested as they did not have an underlying illness. The reality was that flu season was pretty much like every other winter.

As for the backward-walking woman, there was another YouTube clip of her, with the same reporters reporting in the same authoritative tone that she was completely normal. She was either a convincing actor, or had a psychological disorder as opposed to a neurological disorder. They should have just said it like it was; she was probably crazy.

YouTube had, in my eyes anyway, made this complex situation even harder to understand. But the internet isn't all bad. There's always Google, after all …

Google

Google is a mixed blessing. With my modest medical knowledge I feel reasonably capable of filtering out the junk, false hopes, propaganda and outright lies that pervade the internet. But you really have to delve deep to dig out the precious gems of knowledge, and that's why I rarely trust any medical website the students insist I visit.

But Roman insisted I look at the site he had discovered.

'They guarantee a cure,' he said, the excitement in his voice making my gut clench. He leapt into the seat opposite me, and opened his laptop.

You've met Roman before. Earlier that year we diagnosed him with Type I diabetes. He hadn't been coping well.

He placed his laptop on my desk. 'Look, they've got real doctors telling us how it worked for them.' I glanced at some of the endorsements and for a second even I began to hope. There were over thirty testimonials from doctors and other medical types praising the product and claiming they were reducing and even cutting out their insulin altogether, even for Type I diabetics. Without giving the 'secret' away (that would cost a couple of hundred bucks) the testimonials hinted that the special diet and 'approach' to health was revolutionary and life changing.

But I was unconvinced. How could I tell Roman there is no cure for Type I diabetes? But to say nothing would cost him $200, and that's not including the devastation and potential harm these fake cures offer.

The problem with Type I diabetes is that your own immune system has identified the cells that produce insulin as foreign, and attacks them, killing them all off. You physically have no cells left, and there is no other way for your body to produce insulin, which it needs, except by injection.

'You've got to be careful with that online stuff.' I tried to let him down gently. 'There's a lot of conmen out—' He cut me off.

'But the testimonials are from real doctors.'

I've seen fake cures before. For practically every disease known to man, you can find a website offering a cure. I asked him if there was a cure why the rest of the world didn't know about it.

'Because of the money, those corporations ... it even says it right here.' He then showed me the line where it said:

Two new scientific breakthroughs the pharmaceutical companies and health gurus don't want you to know about ...

Roman sat with me as we researched the author of the website and then googled him. We came up with some scary results.

Real reviews from genuine people explained how it was a con, and one reviewer even said that he'd started his own website to counter the lies, but he'd been hit with a very scary letter from a top law firm, telling him to take it down, or prepare for war.

Roman's hopes weren't just dashed; they were ripped to pieces and stomped on. The boy with the needle phobia still had a lifetime of pinpricks in front of him.

The internet is the source of so much misdirection and false hope for those in genuine need – someone like Roman – that it becomes difficult to know who to trust. With so many fraudsters and conmen preying on those who require help and advice, the internet can be a daunting, and frustrating, place for medical practitioners.

The iliac crest?

Molly was a walking, talking, breathing symptom. In the three years I'd known her, she'd grown from a shy little girl to a demanding sixteen-year-old phony, and held the record for most visitations to the health centre; she was a hardened veteran.

Her favourite presentation was the migraine, and she even had a letter from a doctor at home diagnosing her with frequent migraines. But the doctor didn't prescribe any special medicine, and her attacks often coincided with PE, skiing, and bad weather.

The next most common symptom was cramp.

'How would you know, sir, you've never had one,' she always protested when I told her that menstrual cramps are not an illness, but if she didn't feel up to participating in an activity, she would still have to go there and sit and watch. When you say this to most kids, they end up joining in, but Molly wouldn't. She would just sit there, content, her fingers flying across her iPhone.

'She's up to something,' Michaela declared after giving Molly the all clear for the second time in three days. Molly's presentations had become more frequent of late, and I began to wonder if this was part of a bigger plan. But we were worried; there's nothing worse than assuming that just because someone is a regular faker, they're always faking it, and we didn't want to miss anything. So, we referred her to the doctor.

Dr Fritz described her as 'a picture of health', although he did some simple blood tests to give us something concrete. When they came back normal we referred Molly to Cathy, the counsellor, just in case we were missing something psychologically wrong with her.

Cathy didn't hold back. She told Molly that the nurses were tired of her presenting symptoms that never followed any rule, headaches that last one hour, nausea that settled just in time for dinner, cramps that enabled her to pick and choose what activity she wanted. Molly handled the truth like most teenagers – denial, then tears, followed by a promise to improve.

With the school trips coming up, I had been worried that this latest presentation was a tactic to avoid them. As Molly was in the third form, she was set to go on the Outdoor Adventure trip, a physically gruelling hike. It's a compulsory expedition, but there's always some students that attempt to get out of it.

We didn't see Molly for one whole week. For her, that's unheard of, and with the school trip only three weeks away, I thought that maybe I'd misjudged her.

But she came back with a vengeance.

She hobbled into my office, bent in half, her arms crossed over her abdomen. 'It's so bad,' she said, slumping into the chair. If it were anyone else, I would have shown some reaction, and when I didn't respond, she glanced up and added, 'I'm not pretending; it's real this time.'

Teenage logic dictates that admitting you were faking it previously somehow gives more credence to your current situation. I told her to get up on the examination bench.

'Where's it sore?' I began and instead of touching the middle of her stomach like she normally did, her hand brushed the lower right-hand side of her abdomen.

'You've got a sore hip?' I asked, deliberately misinterpreting her, but she shook her head.

'My stomach, the *iliac crest* ...' she dropped the term in casually. 'You're the doctor, you know better than me.' She was close. The words she was looking for were 'right iliac fossa' or the right lower side of the stomach. Pain here automatically sets off alarm bells of suspected appendicitis. Molly was inching towards a self-diagnosis.

If it was her appendix, she needed to go to the hospital straight away, but her choice of words was suspicious. I began my investigation.

She had no fever (an almost-must with appendicitis), but she said she'd had one during the night – plausible.

She had no pain anywhere else; a typical presentation begins with pain around the middle of the stomach, which gradually moves to the right.

Her pulse and blood pressure were fine.

But, of course, I had to be sure.

'We better go to the doctor,' I said, and she was fine with this, but when I added that we might even have to go to the hospital she had a change of heart.

'It's not that bad. I just need some painkillers, that's all.' There was no getting out of this, and I told her that based on her symptoms, we had to see a doctor right away.

'But I don't want one of those camera things,' she said, and I asked her what she meant. 'You know the camera, I saw it online, a ...' she paused, 'the gastric thing ... gastroscopy, that's it. I'm not having that, it looks torture.'

It would be torture if they tried to find her appendix that way. The camera would have to travel through a few feet of intestine. It's not an option; an ultrasound or even CT scan is sometimes used, but often, when the symptoms are obvious, they go straight in and operate.

There are other possible causes for these symptoms. She could be constipated. She could have a UTI (urinary tract infection). But I'm not a doctor, just a nurse.

Dr Fritz ran a number of blood tests, all of which showed no sign of infection or inflammation: an x-ray showed she wasn't constipated, her urine was clear, and she wasn't pregnant. Dr Fritz wasn't convinced it was her appendix, but Molly was unrelenting in her pain and so I took her to hospital.

I last saw Molly as she was wheeled off to theatre. The surgeons weren't convinced, but could find no other explanation. The appendix was normal, but they took it out anyway.

Molly was back at school two days later, lapping up the attention from her friends and teachers. She was tender around the incision sites, but this faded when she found out she would be excused from her trip.

Was Molly faking it? Did she search symptoms online? Well, she virtually admitted as much, but did she realise how far it would go? Sometimes once you commit to a path, there's no turning back, and she may have had an invasive operation she never needed.

Reply all

When it comes to using a computer, unfortunately, I'm not as competent as Molly or most of the other students. However, most everything I do these days is electronic, from writing my notes, sending out appointment schedules, contacting parents or – as Roman and Molly did – researching symptoms and cures. Doing everything online is great when everything goes right, but slip-ups do happen. And the problem with slipping up online is that everyone usually finds out.

I'd recently found a good article giving advice on how to stop smoking and reposted it to the faculty and student body. I often send links to the rest of the school when I find something that I think could be productive. At the very least these articles spark discussion; but this time something different happened.

Shortly after I'd sent the link, I received a new email alert.

Dear sir, I don't mean to be rude, but you're wasting your time.
If we want to stop smoking, we will, but there is nothing you
can say to make us stop.

The email was signed 'Eduard', and the little git hadn't just sent it to me, but to the whole school.

'Who the hell is Eduard?' I just about managed to refrain from instantly replying – such rash responses only tend to exacerbate the situation. Instead, exasperated, I went to Michaela for advice. She had no idea either. Eduard wasn't a regular; he was one of the few kids we did not know.

'Just ignore it,' she suggested, but I couldn't.

'I'm going to do the right thing,' I said, and Michaela shook her head in resignation. 'Oh geez, what you going to do?'

I wanted to be the better person, and to try and help him. He probably expected me to be angry. Instead I replied:

Sorry to hear you feel that way, Eduard, although I'm not so sure everyone thinks the same as you. Perhaps you'd like to come to my office and we can talk about it directly, as emails don't always say what we mean. Perhaps I am wrong, but you sound a bit upset.

I replied to him only, and cut out the rest of school. I got a reply ten minutes later:

I'm sorry sir, but I'm not wasting my time. We will stop when we want to, and not because you think you know what's good for us. You don't know us. You don't know about smoking.

He had posted it all to the whole school, and I was hit with two further emails from students supporting his stance.

There were three emails from teachers on my side, the last of which, from Ms Strawbridge, read: 'What a prick'.

'If he wants war, he's going to get one.' I was pacing about Michaela's office, trying to let off steam. 'Who the hell does he think he is? What good has he done anyone, eh?' Michaela reminded me that I should have let it go. 'Some battles just aren't worth it,' she said. 'You're never going to win this one.'

I did calm down, and I did give up, but not before sending an email to Mr Driscoll, containing the full chain of emails, and the comment, 'I'm not sure he's broken any rules, but he seems pretty angry to me, and his tone is disrespectful. Do you think it's worth having a friendly chat with him?'

'She called him a prick.' The reply came ... but not from Mr Driscoll Ah.

It appeared I hadn't sent the email solely to Mr Driscoll, but to the whole school.

'Ms Strawbridge thinks he's a prick ...' dozens of emails were now joining in.

'That doesn't sound very professional to me.'

'I think he should sue.'

'Instant dismissal, that's what I say.'

'What's a prick?'

'The Oxford English dictionary defines it as ...' This reply listed a dozen definitions, the last of which said '*Slang, derogatory* an obnoxious or despicable man'.

'She can't say that!'

Well, there goes my good deed for the year, and possibly Ms Strawbridge's job. I'd really tried to help, be responsible, be above anger, and be forgiving.

I turned my phone off that night and hid from Ms Strawbridge.

I've stopped posting articles to the whole school. It's just too risky. As for Eduard, well, he had a friendly chat with Mr Driscoll, but suffered no punishment, while Ms Strawbridge was given a gentle reminder about 'being professional' but received no disciplinary action. Meanwhile, the IT department had a horrendous

24 hours trying to remove every trace. Sadly, I'm sure there's a copy somewhere in cyberspace, waiting to bite me, and Ms Strawbridge, in the butt when we least expect it.

Freddy

I don't care what anyone else says, I can't live a lie anymore. I'm coming out the closet. There, I said it. I'm gay.

I hadn't seen this coming for Freddy, but the manner in which he made his announcement was just like him: loud and shocking.

Facebook is a great medium to share your feelings and secrets, no matter how intimate or mundane. I don't think there was another way he could have been more public. Even a YouTube clip of his 'coming-out' would not have been as effective as he had thousands of Facebook friends, each of whom would have told the rest of their friends they 'liked' Freddy's post.

Freddy was no longer one of our students, he was a young man who had recently dropped out of university to pursue a career in acting. I had known him for four years. I wondered how I hadn't seen the signs.

When I'd first met Freddy, he was an annoying little boy.

'He's got ADHD,' his mother had explained when I met them on open day, 'but I don't believe in using drugs.' Freddy hadn't made eye contact with me once, but he wasn't sullen and staring at the ground either. Instead, he was playing with my stethoscope, twiddling with the stationery on my desk, while his ears were plugged into an iPod, his head bopping along to the music.

Should I make him remove them? I wondered. Or should I tell mum to tell her son to remove them? She didn't seem to notice his behaviour, so I asked him to take the headphones off. He didn't say a word, didn't make contact in any noticeable way, his head kept banging along to its own beat. Maybe this was part of his ADHD, but I felt he was trying hard to ignore me.

After my first year of getting to know Freddy, I came to the conclusion that he did not have ADHD because he could concentrate fine when he wanted to and could sit still if needed; he seemed to choose which impulse he was going to act out on. 'I don't have ADHD,' he even told me. 'I'm just passing time.'

Over the years, I got to see how good Freddy was at heart, but also to pick up the pieces when he showed us just how wild and immature he could be, getting drunk while DJ-ing the school prom, for example, or renting an apartment in the village in his name, which the students used as a sex and drinking pad.

Now that he was an adult coming out the closet, I naturally wondered if his rebellious behaviour was a result of conflicting emotions. I sent a reply via Facebook: 'Good on ya, mate. You have to be true to yourself, it's the only way to be happy. PS – always knew you were different.'

I got an instant reply:

'What you mean you knew I was "different"? I didn't write that message. Someone broke into my account and posted it. I'm not gay. I've never been even remotely gay and never will be. I've been fraped.'

Facebook rape, also known as 'frape' (a horrible term if there ever was one), involves someone hijacking your Facebook account and posting messages and statuses in your name.

Well, this was embarrassing, although I wasn't worried because Freddy and I had always got along and always been able to take or give a joke.

Thankfully, Freddy saw the funny side of my mistake in the end. He has kept in contact, and since dropping out of university has begun getting small acting jobs and starred in some commercials. To him, school was just a way of passing time while his real passion was acting. 'When I'm famous I'm going to tell everyone how you always knew I was "different", he likes to remind me.

That was my first experience of 'frape' and I've since been a victim myself.

Fortunately, it wasn't anything as dramatic as announcing I was gay, but I wasn't too keen to be seen to be endorsing 'legal highs' either. I often wonder who was responsible. Secretly, I think it was Freddy having sweet revenge from afar … but it was probably just the wife having a laugh.

Electric friends

When I was young I spent a few years travelling, working my way around the world. This was before Facebook, iPhones, Twitter and the rest of those social media websites, were created. In fact, I think even the internet was pretty new at this time. The best thing about travelling is that you meet so many wonderful people, people that you often share special times with, that your diary becomes full of scribbled, often exotic sounding, names and addresses. It was not electronic, or kept on a smartphone. I had to lug it around in my bag.

I no longer have that address book. I lost it – but it doesn't matter because it no longer had any value. I remember going through it a few years after my time travelling having absolutely no idea who three-quarters of the people were! The quarter that I did remember were people that I still considered friends and who, if I were to contact today, might actually have some interest in catching up.

These days, I've got over 500 Facebook 'friends', but it's the same thing; it's full of people I barely remember and know I will never see again. But 500 is a small number compared to the amount of friends most of my students have.

'I have 2132 friends.' Michelle was in my office because she wanted to be my Facebook friend. 'Why won't you accept my invitation?' I explained that I don't 'friend' current students. 'But why? You've known me for five years. You know me better than anyone, except Mum and Dad.' I asked her if she was FB friends with her parents. 'But you're not my dad, it's different. You're a …' She paused as she tried to find a classification for me. 'You're a, um, well a friend sort of, but not a friend like my normal friends my age.'

'Thanks … I think.'

Not all students considered me their friend; and there were plenty that probably considered me an enemy combatant, but when you spend five years with someone, watching them transform from pimply adolescent to mature young adult, helping them through the typical teenage hurdles, I can see how it can be confusing.

The thing is I'm not their friend, but it's a bit harsh to tell them that directly. Instead, you learn to do it through your interactions with them. Some of the techniques I employ that are guaranteed to subtly get the message across that I'm a 'nurse' or even a 'teacher' – and not their mate – have included:

- Keeping my mobile phone number secret, especially when asked.
- Punishing equally the kids who 'like you' and those who don't.
- Never telling them what I got up to at the weekend, and never asking them, as they may say something I would have to report. They get quite a surprise when you tell them this, but it does actually help reinforce the boundaries.

Michelle was one of the good kids. I had never had to actually use any of the above-mentioned methods with her, and I didn't feel the need to tell her outright that we were not friends.

'It's just not good practice,' I tried to explain. 'It's nothing personal, it's just one of my rules.'

'But other teachers do it. I won't tell anyone. You're one of the good ones. I want to stay in contact.'

I used this moment as an opportunity to remind her about Mr Cosgrove's incident a couple of years ago, and how the internet had nearly cost him his job …

Poor Mr Cosgrove had been flirting with the art teacher in a rather outrageous way. Some rather descriptive messaging had been going back and forth between them for a couple of weeks, which culminated in Mr Cosgrove sending her a picture of his scrotum via his iPhone. The art teacher had loved the picture so much she had put it up on Facebook.

'My balls are on the internet.' Mr Cosgrove had been terrified of the repercussions, while the rest of the faculty had enjoyed making the most of it. The general consensus was that he wouldn't get his balls back.

The laughter stopped when it went viral, well, viral within the student body. The art teacher had forgotten she had accepted friend requests from a couple of students. While technically Mr Cosgrove hadn't done anything wrong, after all it had been between two consenting adults – plus there were no actual identifiable features about whose scrotum it was – and the fact that no name had been attached (it certainly wasn't tagged) he was able to deny that they were actually his. Management were happy to accept this claim and he wasn't fired, although he did voluntarily leave the school at the end of the year, never to return.

Michelle giggled at the memory while I kept a straight face. There are some teachers who let students 'friend' them on Facebook, and Mr Cosgrove had suffered because of it. Since the incident, as well my own personal belief it's simply just a bad idea, I made it a rule never to 'friend' students on Facebook.

It's very touching that some students think so highly of me that they want to be my friend. 'I tell you what. Once you graduate, and you're officially an adult, wait six months and if you still want to be Facebook friends, then I'll accept.' Michelle promised she would do just that.

Six months after graduation, Michelle 'friended' me. We don't actually have any correspondence, which is good. I feel Facebook is just like the diary I kept on my travels. When you're young and impressionable and so many things are new, often unique, and special, it's hard to let go at the time. It's easier to imagine yourself one day catching up and reliving the good memories you had, and refreshing that bond. But, of course, as you get older, it just doesn't happen. To me, Facebook makes it easier to say goodbye, and while in physical terms your farewell is forever, psychologically you'll always have that electronic link that keeps you connected

CHAPTER FIVE

Drugs

Getting your buzz on

Every year there's usually a handful of children who test positive for drugs, usually marijuana, but there are other ways to get high besides taking pills or smoking something green.

One Monday afternoon I received an emergency call to go to the school gym because a child was unconscious. The child was awake by the time I arrived, but over the next month another six kids passed out. 'It's a game,' Rich confided in me one day and I asked him to explain. Rich was in his graduating year of school and I'd known him for five years and he had become a great source of student gossip. I know he didn't tell me everything because he wasn't an informer, and he never told me any names, but he did keep me in the loop about any potentially dangerous behaviour.

'They make themselves pass out, or at least come close to it.' I naturally asked why. 'The head-rush is pretty intense.' I asked him if he'd tried it and he admitted that he had tried it once. 'I just wanted to see if it was actually possible. I didn't believe you could really do it.' He hadn't done it again, as it had made him sick to the stomach and he'd thrown up, but according to him 'everyone's doing it'.

The technique is simple:

- Squat down against a wall
- Take in 20–30 deep breaths rapidly
- Take one last deep breath, hold it and stand up
- Keep holding till your vision clears (that's if you haven't blacked out by then)
- Get someone to catch you

This craze died out after a couple of months, but not before we saw another half-dozen potential head injuries.

Just like I can't keep up with every new fad, or way of getting a buzz, I can't possibly keep in the loop about every new drug that comes on the scene, particularly when so many of them aren't even classified yet, and as a result are not illegal, but are equally (if not more) dangerous as the known stuff. The kids were once so desperate to try something new, they started swallowing nutmeg. Who would have thought that such a harmless ingredient could give such a powerful trip? There's no way to test for nutmeg intoxication, but it was popular for at least six months. The kids would swallow whole bottles of the stuff, often with warm milk, and they'd be high for up to 24 hours. The come-down was never good, but are they ever?

The most recent crazes, as of 2014, were the 'bed bugs' and 'beeswax lip balm' highs. I only found out about these because a couple of senior girls asked me if I'd heard of them, and if they really worked. After a bit of research I discovered that, apparently, putting a certain lip balm on your eyelids gives you a drunken feeling. The only ingredients in it are beeswax, vitamin E and peppermint. I hoped none our kids got it in their eyes as this would really hurt. I'm not convinced this will make you feel drunk, although you may get watering eyes and blurred vision.

As for smoking crushed bed bugs, my first question was 'who the hell finds these things out?' and 'where the hell are the kids going to get bed bugs from?' As much as the kids love to moan about their rooms, we haven't had bed bugs yet.

It turned out the bed bug myth had begun as an April Fools' joke that had become a viral hit and lasted a lot longer than just one day. If any of our students did manage to find some bed bugs, or any kind of bug to smoke, then more power to them. Besides, it's not exactly something we could test for, I think. Although there are plenty of substances we can and do.

A *testing time*

I had never expected monitoring kids for drugs to be part of my role as a school nurse. I do feel conflicted at times when testing students because a positive result means instant expulsion. It's a view Michaela and Justine share with me. We're the ones the students are supposed to turn to for help; we're not supposed to be involved in getting them kicked out of school.

They say that absolute power corrupts absolutely, but a more accurate description would be to say that power corrupts most other people – but not me. It just makes me nervous. It would have been much easier if I had been given a random list of names, instead of being told to choose whomever I felt like.

'I need six done today,' Mr Driscoll had explained. 'We need to be seen to be making an effort.' He then stressed that the purpose of drug testing is not to catch anyone out; instead he wants to discourage anyone from taking them in the first place. Choosing students at random is not as easy as it sounds, especially when you must have a mix of boys and girls, new and returning, as well as someone who has been tested before because 'They have to see that it's random, and just because they've been tested once, doesn't mean they won't be tested again.'

These non-random criteria neatly ruled out the only way I knew of picking someone at random, which was to close my eyes and point at a name on a list. There was no way it could be random, because I now had to pick and choose whom to test, which sort of defeats the purpose. It also doesn't help that names and faces began to surface in my mind, but I had a job to do and, thankfully, I came up with a solution. I chose Mr Wright's class because he had one of the biggest classes on campus, with about twenty-five students, and so was most likely to meet the needed criteria.

'I need some volunteers,' I said as I stood in the doorway and Mr Wright kindly volunteered them all, but no one offered. Instead they looked at me suspiciously. I would have to pick. Should I choose someone like Chris, simply because he fits a certain profile? He's never tested positive, but was the stereotypical surfer dude from California with the long blonde hair, skateboard and chin fluff. He was a good kid, with good grades whose family I had come to know over the years as I'd looked after his older sister and brother. I didn't want to choose him because I was worried he might fail, but now I couldn't discard him completely because that was not the random thing to do.

I chose Chen because he was Asian and looked the academic type, surely not a smoker. Next were the two Canadians, Laura and Rob, although I was a bit nervous about choosing Rob because all the Canadian male friends I had known over the years were into smoking pot. Then came two unreadable Russians, one male and one female and both new. That left one student to choose who had been tested before, which meant I reluctantly picked Chris.

'Dude, that's not fair,' Chris moaned. He insisted he wasn't worried, but angry because he was being singled out for looking like a stoner. 'It's the principle,' he said, and perhaps he was right.

'Sorry mate, got no choice,' I said as I explained I simply needed someone who had been tested before, and he was the only one in the class I had randomly selected. They sat in the health centre sipping water, waiting for the urge to pee. Chris asked for a second glass because he couldn't go, while the two Russians went first and were given the all-clear. Chen went next, followed by the two Canadian students, but Chris still couldn't pee.

The longest I normally have to wait is about fifteen minutes, but Chris still hadn't been after twenty minutes. 'It's not my fault, I went just before you came and got me.' I hoped this was true and reminded him that the kidneys produce 1ml of urine a minute.

'I'm not dumb enough to do pot here,' he said irritably. 'I'm over that sort of shit. I just don't need a piss.' I ignored the bad language and instead asked him what he meant by being 'over that sort of shit'.

'If I was back in California, it wouldn't be a big deal. Everyone's tried it. I get offered pot all the time at school, but I don't do it anymore. I did it a bit in ninth and tenth grade, but I'm over it. If I want to get high, I'll wait till I get back home. But I won't, because like I said, I don't do that shit. And besides, you really think I'm stupid enough to waste 100,000 euros getting kicked out of school? My dad would kill me.'

Another twenty minutes passed before he was ready to pee. 'Enjoy,' he said as he passed me his sample before heading back to class. I stopped him at the door to ask if he wanted to see the test, as every student, even the innocent ones, is eager to see the physical result. He shrugged his shoulders and asked 'why' before heading out the door.

His test was clear.

You shouldn't judge anyone by the way they look, but it's only natural – we all do it to some degree or another. However, I've been caught out, and had the most innocent looking faces test positive for the most surprising of drugs.

There was the Saudi royal who tested positive for heroin, then the bookish, serious looking Chinese sisters who not only had great grades, but the strongest positive result for cocaine I've ever seen. There was also the quiet first timer who had the misfortune to be caught in the act. And then there's Jimmy …

Jimmy

Jimmy wasn't exactly 'hanging out' in the health centre. He had been referred to me because other students, as well as staff, had heard him tell others how much he smoked. Several teachers described him as sounding proud of it.

Jimmy had transferred to our school from a public school in California and it was his first time in Europe, but not his first time away from home. 'I can't believe you can grow your own pot, dude, it's awesome,' he said by way of greeting, referring to the lax laws in this part of Europe. I told him that it's not appropriate to talk about such habits out loud because 'it's not cool' but he didn't get the hint.

'Dude, everyone smokes it. My little brother even smokes it.'

It's hard to figure out the number of students that smoke pot, but every year there are at least two or three that get expelled for taking drugs. Unlike most others his age, Jimmy didn't try hiding the fact that he smoked, and even explained that his parents were worried about his habit. At eighteen years of age, he had been smoking for the last four years, and his parents wanted him as far away as possible from the drug problems they had there. So they sent him to an isolated school high up in the Alps.

Jimmy's rationale for using pot was the usual: it's harmless, everyone does it, and it's medicinal. 'As soon as I get back to L.A., I'm getting my pot licence. I ain't never gonna stop.'

With marijuana so entrenched in his way of thinking, I couldn't see Jimmy lasting long at our school. 'You do realise that we do drug testing here?' I explained, but he just shrugged his shoulders: 'What will be, man. I'll try and be good, but I can't make any promises.'

'Your parents spent a lot of money to send you here. Are you just going to throw that money away?' I told him, but it fell on deaf ears. Jimmy wasn't the slightest bit put out. 'That's just a drop in the ocean. My parents wouldn't even notice.' His family may not notice the money (rumour had it his family had recently bought an island) but his habit was affecting his life as he was failing high school and had been uprooted from his friends and sent to live in a foreign speaking country, but he couldn't see this, or chose to ignore it.

'It's probably not a good idea to tell everyone about your habit, you should learn to be discreet. You're going to run out of schools to take you.'

Jimmy explained that he had been kicked out of three previous schools. The first had been a private day school.

'And this doesn't bother you?' He shrugged his shoulders and said it wasn't his fault because if his mother hadn't found the pot he'd hidden in an old shoe in his wardrobe then he would have been fine.

'What sort of mum looks in such places?' he said, sounding almost nostalgic. He laughed when I told him that he wasn't the first to think that old shoes were great hiding places, and that mothers are great at cleaning in the most obscure corners of their child's bedroom.

After being withdrawn from his first school, he'd been sent to a private boarding school in the States. He hadn't fared any better, his grades again dropped, and he'd failed a random drug test.

Jimmy's parents had become tired of throwing away money on expensive institutions and desperate to get their child on the right track, but nothing seemed to work. They then tried the public school system where it was tough, and surely he'd learn to appreciate just how privileged he was, and see the error of his ways. But public school was no different. 'It was easy to fit in,' he said, because 'it's the easiest place in the world to get some gear'.

When everyone became aware that nothing had changed, his mother had told me via email that we were his last chance. He had to clean his act up, or they would be taking drastic action. I replied, telling her that I felt her son needed more than we could offer, but she still wanted to give our school a try.

'Why should I hide who I am? It's part of me. If people don't like it, that's their problem.' Jimmy sounded insulted at my suggestion he should be discreet.

'Marijuana is who you are? Great to see you aiming so high in life.' I was getting annoyed at his apathetic attitude to everything, although this was no surprise. Teenagers can be the most stubborn people in the world at the best of times, let alone with the brain-numbing effects of drugs. Jimmy didn't react to my insult, probably because it went way over his head.

'Your mum said this is your last chance.' She had repeated this phrase often, although never explained what she exactly meant. 'Do you even give a damn?'

Jimmy fired up. 'You don't know me, of course I give a damn.'

'Then will you at least make an effort? A genuine attempt to stay in school, and follow the rules? For your family's sake.'

Something flashed in Jimmy's eyes at the mention of his parents. And I realised, he wasn't a bad guy, just a naïve kid. After a bit more cajoling, Jimmy left my office promising to 'see what he could do'. He almost sounded sincere. But, ultimately, he needed more help than me or the school could provide. Four months later Jimmy's drug test came back positive for marijuana and he was asked to leave the school.

Many schools take on children who need more than they can offer, especially private schools as they have a pretty big financial incentive to make it work. The powers that be often genuinely believe they can provide the structure and support for children, but it's not always the case. I shouldn't be so cynical, 'everyone needs a second chance, a blank slate,' as Mr Driscoll often says.

Mr Driscoll is partially right as I've seen students with bad attitudes come good in the end, but it's more to do with luck and chance as anything else, regardless of how much effort we put in.

Thankfully, for Jimmy, it wasn't the end.

Parents don't want their children to go through the hardships they experienced, and as such it's hard as a parent to deny your child the things privilege and money can buy, especially when you are denying them the things that you've worked so hard for.

But that is exactly what Jimmy's parents did.

They cut him off, and kicked him out the house. But not before finding him a job as a trainee chef. They told him that once he finished, and was financially independent, they would consider sharing their wealth with him once again. I saw Jimmy a couple of years later when he returned to visit the school. He'd come to the Alps to ski, and he was allowed on campus to catch up with anyone who had got to know him in his short time here. I was one of a dozen or so staff who remembered him.

'It's strange being back,' he mused. He was sitting in my office, in the same seat where I'd lectured him before, drinking in the view out my window. 'It's so small,' he said, referring to the school, not the mountains around us. 'You think you know it all. You think nothing else matters other than getting high.'

This was a different Jimmy to the one I knew before. There were the physical changes: the work had done him good, his body had filled out, and he had muscles where he used to be skin and bone. But it was his tempered thoughts, his sharp observations that made him all grown up.

'Do you still smoke?' I asked.

'Not really, not with the job,' he confessed. 'Pot and eighteen hour shifts don't really go well together.' He flashed a smile. This may be the new and improved Jimmy, but the fun lad was still inside. He explained he does still have the odd toke now and then, but the smoking is an occasional break from his reality, instead of being his reality.

I'll never forget his parting comment. 'It's good to have a clear head.'

I think Jimmy has to be one of the luckiest guys around. Not only does he have the security of wealth, but he also has parents who are brave enough to make painful decisions for the wellbeing of their son. I wish all parents were able to do this.

Ruben's demons

If we only had to worry about marijuana, things may not be so bad, but there's a whole world of dangerous substances out there, many of which I only find out about when things break.

He had armed himself with a frying pan and was warning me to stay away. Even unarmed, any patient in this state can be deadly, and while a frying pan might not seem like much of a weapon, it could easily fracture my skull. But I couldn't stay too far away; someone had to keep him in sight until backup arrived.

No one would believe me if I told them just how frightening and even dangerous nursing can be. If I was twenty years younger perhaps I would have tried something rash, like disarm the kid. He was only sixteen years old. I'm almost forty and I should be able to handle him, but with age comes caution.

I've seen the boys punching and kicking the bag in the gym and thought to myself 'I could still take him'. You remember your glory days when you felt ten foot tall and invincible. When you're surrounded by teenagers, it's common to think you're still fitter, faster and smarter than the lot of them. Being clever and more experienced does count, but I was brought sharply back to reality when I saw how angry, frightened and big Ruben was.

Ruben had only been with us for four months, but I still couldn't believe I had not seen any signs; these types of problems usually build up over time.

'They've poisoned me!' he kept muttering to himself, although I suspected most likely in response to the voices in his head. 'Don't make me use this. Are you one of them?' I shook my head.

'I'm not one of them,' I replied as calmly as possible. I didn't try to find out exactly who or what 'one of them' was, but I delved into his delusion a little, to make sure to differentiate myself from 'the ones' that had 'poisoned' him. It could be his teachers, the dorm staff, or everyone on campus.

I reached one hand into my pocket. 'What you doing?' He took a step towards me and I quickly removed my hand.

'Just calling a friend, that's all. Will you let me call a friend? I promise he's not "one of them". He's a good guy.'

Ruben didn't respond straight away, he looked confused, he wanted help, but didn't know who to trust.

'You can trust me, Ruben. You've seen me before, in the health centre. Remember I helped you when you were sick.' Ruben lowered the frying pan, and reluctantly agreed to let me make the call. 'You promise not to bring the bad people?' I promised him I'd only bring people I trusted.

Soon the headmaster and the school counsellor were heading our way.

As they approached, Mr Driscoll took one look at the armed teenager, his agitated movements, his big searching eyes, and stopped behind me, quietly asking what was going on. Cathy, the counsellor, kept calm, waiting for me to take the lead.

I introduced the new arrivals to Ruben – 'You remember Mr Driscoll?' Ruben nodded his head. 'And this is Cathy, she works with me in the health centre. They're both good people. You can trust them.' Ruben wasn't so ready to trust them, but he said they could stay, as long as they didn't come any closer. They reassured him that they would stay where they were.

We needed the police and paramedics, but we also needed to get Ruben to a place where he couldn't easily flee. The paramedics would be at least 45 minutes away, while the local police officer (if he was on call that night) could be another twenty minutes away. Fortunately it was a cold December night, and I decided to use the pretext of needing to stay warm to convince him to come inside.

'I'm not going anywhere with you. It's a trap.'

To gain his trust I said I'd give him my key to the building and let him lead the way to the cafeteria. Cathy and Mr Driscoll continued to let me take the lead. Mr Driscoll probably realised he was out of his depth, while Cathy was experienced enough to sit back and let the person whom Ruben trusted continue to take charge.

'There's more than one way out of the cafeteria,' I explained, 'you won't be trapped. You can leave anytime.' I placed the key on the ground and stepped back. Ruben quickly scooped it up, his eyes keeping us in sight the whole time. We followed him into the empty dining hall.

I used this distraction and asked Cathy to call the paramedics, while asking Mr Driscoll to get some male staff to come and stand outside the cafeteria, but to stay out of sight.

Ten minutes later we were seated around a table, Ruben resting the frying pan in front of him.

Should I tell him that the paramedics were on their way? He may feel betrayed and bolt, or strike, or go completely berserk. I've only dealt with psychiatric patients in the controlled environment of a ward, and even then I've seen some pretty hairy stuff, but now I was beginning to appreciate just how hard it was to remain in control, especially when you're the one everyone else is turning to for guidance.

'You think you've been poisoned?' I had an idea I hoped would work.

'It's the food. It's something in the food.' He was eager to talk about this.

'Why don't you let us take you to hospital then to make sure?' I explained. 'They could test and see if you've been poisoned. They could help.' To my relief Ruben agreed upon this course of action. 'I'll go and order an ambulance, will that be OK?' Ruben nodded his head.

Within the hour the paramedics arrived with two police officers. As the village only has one officer living on the mountain, they'd obviously brought backup from the valley. After a hurried conversation in the corridor the police agreed to stay out of sight while the paramedics followed me in to see Ruben.

Ruben agreed to leave the frying pan behind, and Cathy went with him in the ambulance to the hospital.

Ruben spent three days in hospital, where he improved dramatically. He calmed down and even said he was only joking about being poisoned – although that's a worrying sign in itself – but his parents had arrived to take him home.

It was too soon for a diagnosis, and he'd have to go endure a lot of tests to rule out physical causes for his problem, before taking things to the next level. He was discharged into the care of his parents and flown back to Canada.

Several months later pieces of the puzzle began to slot in place. Cathy kept in contact with Ruben's mother, and we found out he'd been inhaling spice, also known as synthetic cannabis.

It may sound an incredibly brave thing to admit to, but after two weeks in a psychiatric unit he simply wanted to go home and didn't want to be labelled a schizophrenic or in his own words 'a nutter'. He does not have a diagnosis of schizophrenia but he cannot touch drugs again, or he may end up with one. Spice has been the most common synthetic cannabis I've seen, although other brands I've come across are K2, Atomic bomb, Funky Monkey and 8Ball … the list goes on, as does the damage. It's described as synthetic cannabis, but with a few extra branches attached to the chemical formula, making it unidentifiable. If a particular brand gets banned because it's proven to be harmful, they just tweak it a little more, bringing it back into the 'unidentified substance' category and making it legal again.

If you try googling the different brands of synthetic cannabis, you'll find hundreds to choose from. From what I can see, the synthetic stuff is especially dangerous because it's an unknown, it's an uncategorised chemical substance of which we don't know the exact effects – there is no way to know how someone will react. It's also scary because we can't test for it because the moment a successful test comes out, the manufacturers tweak the formula to beat the system yet again.

Drug manufacturers are adept at staying one step ahead of the system, unlike our students, who get themselves into a right mess. Take Kate and Kelly for example …

Kate and Kelly

Kate was at least honest about being dishonest, but one day that honesty was going to get her in trouble, not to mention put me in an exquisitely difficult position.

Kate and Kelly visited me nearly every day, usually to say hello, share some gossip, or fish for some. Both girls were sixteen, but already smart. Kate wanted to be a doctor, Kelly wanted to study chemistry and pharmaceuticals.

'I'm going to cure cancer,' Kelly had once declared. Not to be outdone, Kate had said she was going to be a brain surgeon. I wished them well.

'We're not sick, just tired.' Kate's confession lacked remorse, but her enthusiasm was contagious. 'Please excuse us for one hour, just this class, that's all,' Kate pleaded as she dropped to her knees, hands clasped in front of her. Kelly followed her; the two were twins, inseparable. If one was going to miss class, then both were.

'Up you get girls, you'll be late for drama class,' I mocked. The melodramatic antics were not disturbing, but the fact they really expected me to excuse them from class, was.

'We don't do drama,' Kate replied, but quickly cottoned on when I suggested she'd do well in Hollywood.

'Did we tell you you're the best nurse?'

Maybe they thought of me as an ally, even a friend. I knew that if that were the case, I needed to set them right. But have I mentioned what a pushover I can be?

The girls skipped to class, with a note from me excusing them for being ten minutes late.

It was the very last week of school when Kate sent me an email.

'Urgent, please help, can you call me or Kelly?'

They hadn't called the emergency number to get the nurse on call, which means it's probably something sensitive and personal, which usually translated to: pregnancy, STD, or in need of emergency contraceptive. I gave Kate a call.

'We're sorry' were Kate's first words. To which I said, 'It's OK, just tell me what's wrong.'

'Do you think they'll drug test us?' Kate asked, and I suddenly felt sick.

The previous year Mr Driscoll had insisted on testing many of the seniors in their last week of school. This had come about because there had been a lot of rumours circulating about large numbers of students taking legal highs. Our tests cannot detect these, but he had wanted to set an example. It seemed, rumours had arisen that the same tests would be carried out this year.

'I can't answer that, Kate, you should know that. What have you taken?' She confessed that she and Kelly had smoked some marijuana that morning.

'Please sir, we're really sorry, we screwed up; we won't do it again. You're not going to tell on us, are you?'

I wasn't going to tell on them, although I explained that this was not because I'm a friend, but because as a nurse I can't discuss something I've been told in confidence.

The girls were young women who would soon likely go to university, able to do what they liked, with whom they liked, whenever they felt the urge. Was this a one-off lapse? How long had they been smoking? Was it their first time? I asked Kate …

'I've been good, I haven't done it all year,' she promised.

'Ah, Kate, are you telling me that you smoked when you were fifteen?'

'Well, um, fourteen actually, but not a lot, just a couple of times.'

When I asked her about the risks of smoking pot at such a young age, she said it's harmless. When I asked her if she'd tried anything else, she admitted to trying ecstasy, 'but only once, just half a tablet'. She was surprised to hear me say that ecstasy is also dangerous.

And these were the doctors of tomorrow, supposedly.

Kate and Kelly needed help. They needed to be educated. They needed to know that there are risks involved, and I arranged a meeting with them and Cathy.

It's moments like these when you realise how powerful an influence you have on the people in your care. Why did Kate and Kelly feel they could turn to me? What was the right thing to do? At the very least I could make them educated drug users; often that's more productive than just telling them to 'Say no'.

Somehow, so many intelligent, well-raised kids think that taking drugs is normal, and safe because 'everyone does it'. That may be the case, sadly, but how can we stop this vicious cycle? I only wish I knew. My job would be a lot easier if I did.

CHAPTER SIX

Counselling

Ameena

I'm a good nurse when it comes to the physical side of things – the cuts, bruises, breaks and illnesses. But a big part of being a nurse to so many school children is dealing with cases that are psychological, emotionally very delicate and private. We do have a counsellor in the staff to deal with these types of issues, but our roles often overlap, as our resources are stretched paper-thin.

Most of the counselling I do is anything but specialised. But by simply being there listening and helping people get along, hopefully it all helps …

As the only Saudi female at school, Ameena was unique. Oh, there were plenty of Saudi boys, drinking, partying and chasing women during extravagant weekend trips to the big cities in the valley, but in a lot of Saudi families women tend to be kept close to home. I suspect the only reason Ameena was allowed to come to boarding school was because she had two older brothers who could look after her.

At fifteen years of age Ameena was not just a couple of years younger than her nearest brother, she was the opposite of her brothers. While the boys were loud, funny, flash with cash and indifferent about school work, Ameena was softly spoken, kind, thoughtful and reserved. She was near the top of her class in all her subjects. But it wasn't this that made her really stand out.

It was the first week back at school following the Christmas break, and several teachers had been in contact with me to say that they were concerned about Ameena. They told me she seemed sad and not her usual happy self, and when she finally broke into tears during class, she was sent to see me.

Tearful female teenagers are not my speciality, and with her being a tearful teenage female from Saudi, I felt I was not the right person to comfort her. Whether this conclusion was right or wrong, ignorant or intuitive, I meant well. I was just trying to take into consideration her cultural values. But I needn't have worried.

What does one say to a crying female Saudi teenager? You keep your mouth shut and offer her a box of tissues, and wait.

'It's not fair,' she finally said, once her tears had dried.

'What's not fair?'

She didn't respond; she suddenly looked worried. 'It's nothing.' I reminded her that it obviously wasn't 'nothing' or she wouldn't be in tears. I thought it the right time to tell her that several of her teachers had been concerned about her.

'You don't have to tell me. Sometimes a big cry is all you need,' I said.

She slowly shook her head, before seeming to make up her mind.

'You won't tell my brothers or my parents I'm here, will you?' I said I wouldn't tell her brothers, but said I couldn't promise not to tell her parents if I thought her health was in danger.

'Oh, I'm not in any danger, although my parents would be very angry.'

I was trying to figure out what could be wrong. 'If it's about boys, and, you know, private stuff, I'm not allowed to tell your parents, so don't worry.'

'Oh my goodness' – her face turned red – 'it's nothing like that. My parents would be way beyond angry if it was anything like that.' I felt immensely relieved. A pregnant teenage Saudi was not something I would be well equipped to handle.

'I do have a friend though, a female friend …' She hesitated, unsure if she should continue. She took a deep breath, seeming to make up her mind.

'It's Adina,' she said, as if this explained everything.

'Ah … I see … And why is that a problem?' I asked, my lips working before my mind had processed the implications of her announcement.

She shook her head. 'I knew you wouldn't understand.'

I asked her to help me understand.

'Well, you do know she's Jewish, right?' I didn't know she was Jewish, or care for that matter, but Ameena said she'd been worrying about this ever since they'd become friends. A recent trip home during the Christmas break had reminded her of the risk she was taking.

'Do you know what I've been taught all my life by my family?' I shook my head. I already sensed I was about to learn a life lesson, an insight that would change my view of the world. 'I've been raised to hate Jews, but I don't think I hate them.' Ameena paused briefly while I tried to digest what I had been told. 'It's just the way it is where I'm from, I don't know what to do.'

I had never been raised to hate anybody. I can't imagine parents deliberately poisoning the minds of their offspring, although I'm sure the family do not see it that way.

I know her brothers – along with many other Saudi students – and I like them. They're nice guys who seem normal. That is, they're capable of kindness, compassion, and empathy. I asked what her brothers would do if they found out.

She wasn't sure, but felt that they might feel obligated to tell her parents. 'They're not like your average Saudi,' she added. She was right. The drinking, womanising lads were not your typical image of a Saudi Arabian. 'Do they hate Jewish people?' I asked, referring to her brothers.

She smiled at my question. 'They don't hate anyone, but they'll do what they think they have to, especially if it involves their little sister. They may say something to protect me from bad influences.'

In college we talked about cultural sensitivity and learning how to avoid accidentally offending someone from another culture. I have to confess that at the time I thought it was a load of rubbish. I'm not sure how you accidentally offend someone, because with a bit of tolerance on both sides, and some honest communication, you can usually resolve most issues. But this problem was beyond anything I'd ever come across. I was venturing into new territory, and I didn't want to take a bad step that would affect both of us negatively.

'Are you sure none of them know?'

She shook her head. It seems that between the parties, drinking and women chasing, her brothers weren't keeping all that close an eye on their little sister.

'What do you want from me? How can I help?' She shrugged her shoulders, not sure what to say.

'It's good to talk,' she eventually said.

'Are you going to stay friends?'

She shrugged. 'I guess.'

'Good.'

When I look back at our conversation, I had done nothing miraculous, I had barely said anything, but Ameena left my office a little happier than when she'd come in. Often being someone to talk to, a safe outlet for the kids to vent their worries or frustrations is all it takes to be able to help.

Through conversations like this, I began to appreciate just how special my boarding school was. If someone like Ameena could make friends with a supposed enemy, and if the other nationalities and religions could co-exist peacefully, despite the way they had been raised, then perhaps these children could be one of the last generations to continue thinking the same as past generations. Time will tell, I suppose, but in Ameena's eyes at least, there is hope.

Rocket man

Sometimes religion, culture and power all look the same to me. Some will fight for one, or all, of these reasons, others will fight not really having a grasp of any of them.

At fifteen years of age, Faisal was ready to fight for his cause, although right now, he was trying to convince me his black eye was the result of an accident with a door. But I knew better. I've seen hundreds of black eyes, and Faisal's colourful face was the result of a punch-up. It also helped that I had been told by some of his teachers exactly why he'd started a fight.

The eyeball seemed fine. No visual changes, no pain, and although the white of the eye was bloodshot, Faisal was lucky – because the rest of the eye socket was badly swollen, black and blue.

'Don't insult me, Faisal,' I said as I explained just how many black eyes I'd seen. He shrugged his shoulders. 'Sorry, sir, I didn't mean to give offence, but I did walk into a door.'

I was nearing the halfway point of my second year at the school and I'd got to know Faisal pretty well by this stage. He was one of the easy-going kids who would often wander into the health centre and try to distract me for twenty minutes with an interesting story, gossip, or show genuine interest in my background and home country. Because of this, I felt that we had a good rapport.

In fact, a lot of the kids who had been at school for more than a year had developed a good working relationship with the nursing staff. Many come to my office just to talk. Sometimes it can be health related, but just as often I can find myself talking politics, religion, business, anything their young minds could think of.

I wasn't going to let it rest there with Faisal. This wasn't his first fight and I wanted it to be his last, no matter how unlikely that was. Faisal was a dedicated warrior in his own private religious war, and had been heard in class telling everyone 'you're going to hell' if they didn't surrender to Allah. I may not be able to change his views, but I just might be able to help him control his anger. I didn't need a confession from him to be able to help.

Faisal was grinning. I was disappointed he didn't seem to be taking this seriously. I've been in my fair share of punch-ups, although I'd never actually started one. Faisal was going to graduate soon and he needed to learn that in the adult world, a punch-up was treated a lot more seriously.

'Well, it's none of my business anyway, Faisal. Fortunately your eye looks like it is going to be fine … this time,' I said, before adding: 'Is it true?'

He looked confused.

'What're you talking about?'

'Well, I heard a rumour about you. I probably shouldn't say.'

Faisal leaned towards me, his face suddenly serious, insisting I tell him what the rumour was.

I was treading a very dangerous line, but I've always felt boundaries are there to be pushed. This wasn't so much a rumour, but it was what people had been saying to him to get a reaction.

'I heard that you're half Jewish.'

Faisal jumped out of his char, and stood over me, fuming. 'Who said that?'

I shrugged my shoulders, a forced smile on my lips. 'I'm just kidding, Faisal. I wanted to see how you'd react.'

My smile vanished as I realised I might have gone too far.

'If you weren't a teacher, I'd hit you right now.' Faisal was deadly serious, but there was no turning back for me now.

'Don't you see what you've done, Faisal?'

He grunted a reply, his hands clenching and unclenching at his sides. I felt my own ire rising in frustration.

'I know you're not Jewish.'

'Why'd you say it then? There's some things you don't joke about.'

'If you sit and listen, maybe you'll learn why.' He reluctantly returned to his seat, his hands clutching the armrests.

Faisal is from Lebanon, and the tensions between Israel and Hezbollah had been reaching new heights (even though to my relative ignorance they seem to be in a permanent state of tension), although everyone would still be surprised about the breakout of full-scale war in the upcoming months.

I was never going to be able to make him change his views on who to like and dislike, and it's not really my job to do so, but if I could make him see what was happening to him and the way he was perceived at the school, something good could come from this. Faisal had been known to get pretty fired up if someone even joked about him being Jewish.

'You're reacting exactly the way I expect; you're so predictable. I know what buttons to push.' Faisal's face was a blank, registering neither understanding nor confusion, and definitely not forgiveness. 'The kids want to see you react. They want to see you get in a fight. Have you thought that maybe they want to see you get in trouble? You're playing right into their hands.'

There was some softening in Faisal's aura, time to drive the message home. 'Nobody wants a troublemaker around. I could push your buttons to make you do something that would get you in big trouble, maybe I could get you kicked out of school.'

Most of the kids Faisal was fighting with couldn't care less what nationality or religion he was. They simply enjoyed watching him get fired up.

'Stop acting like a head case.'

'What did you just call me?' he asked, surprised instead of angry.

I can't say I've ever called a student a 'head case' before; immediately I realised I probably should try to avoid doing so again. I'd lost control of the conversation. But I didn't feel like a teacher anymore, or even a nurse, just an older human being who has lived a bit, trying to get through to a decent lad.

'You're like a puppet. I can pull on your string and watch you jump. There are people in this school who know how to make you dance to their tune. Am I getting through to you? Stop being their bitch.'

'You can't say that.' He was right, I can't. What was wrong with me? 'Too late.'

'OK … I get it all right, I get it. I've heard enough.' The Faisal I knew was returning. 'I've never thought of it like that before,' he added, before admitting that he was still disturbed at being called a 'head case'.

'You have to see that you're only harming yourself. If you get in one more fight, you're out of school … for good. Don't be a victim.'

We sat in silence for a full minute (which is pretty long for a teenager) while he worked out what to do from here. His reaction caught me by surprise as he stood up and shook my hand.

'Does this mean you're going to refrain from reacting to everyone who pushes your buttons?' He said he was willing to give it a try.

Faisal finished the school year without getting into any more fights. It was during the last week of school he told me that when he stopped reacting, people eventually gave up provoking him.

Unfortunately, stories like this don't always have happy endings. During the school summer break war broke out between Israel and Hezbollah and upon Faisal's return to school he confided to me that he'd been spent his time working for Hezbollah.

'I wanted to fire the rockets, but they said I was too young.' Faisal didn't seem so young anymore, but I couldn't reconcile the image of such an easy-going, likeable, intelligent and, ultimately, good young man aspiring to be a rocket-launching soldier. 'But they let me work as a messenger boy,' Faisal added proudly.

I knew I would not be able to make him change his views and it's not my job to choose sides. There's over fifty nationalities represented at my school, so it pays not to. I like to think that I at least helped him learn to control his anger, and learn not to be controlled by others, but when I look at the bigger picture, I'm probably being naïve.

It's strange, because Faisal is a good person with a good heart. It's strange because I know students, and friends, on both sides of this conflict and I wonder how can two people on opposing sides of a conflict both have a good heart and kind nature? I struggle to find a 'bad guy'.

Niko

Niko wasn't a bad guy. In fact, he was a lot like Faisal, a regular kid with deep-rooted convictions.

As usual Niko had forgotten to collect his daily medication, and I went in search of him, eventually cornering him as he waited outside the headmaster's office.

'What'd you do this time?'

'Nothing.'

'Well, you can tell me more about this thing you didn't do on the way to the health centre.'

His meeting with the headmaster would have to wait because he hadn't received any medicines for three days and his health took priority.

Niko had recently been diagnosed with epilepsy and was struggling to adjust to his new life.

Niko was struggling because he could no longer drink alcohol.

'There's no such thing as a Pole who doesn't drink vodka.' He truly believed what he said, but he also knew that alcohol and his epilepsy medication should never mix. Such prescriptions mixed with alcohol can actually have the opposite effect and increase the likelihood of seizures occurring, as well as the

243

severity. His solution was to stop taking his tablets when he planned to drink.

It's hard for any teenager to be told they can't do something, and being told you can't drink when all your friends do quite regularly is extra tough. But Niko's life could depend on him following these instructions. Maybe he didn't believe us, or perhaps I simply did not appreciate how much pressure Niko felt in order to fit in.

I asked him why he was waiting to see the headmaster, and he insisted that he hadn't done anything. 'Mr Currie sent me for no reason. I didn't do anything wrong.' Mr Currie was an old hand and kept his classes in line, and it was a little unusual for him to send someone to Mr Driscoll.

'What were you doing just before you were asked to leave?'

'We were talking about gays …'

Niko was a nice kid with a warm heart. This was going to be difficult to hear …

'I said I hate them.'

Lots of teenage boys talk like this and I want to believe it's more habit than actual hate. His comments weren't as bad as some I've heard in my time, but that's little consolation.

'Do you know anyone who is gay?' I enquired.

He shook his head.

'It's unnatural. It's a disease. We need to get rid of them.' His words sounded rehearsed, learned, and lacked malice. Did he really think it a disease?

'Should we get rid of people with epilepsy then? That's a disease.' He flinched as if struck. So cruel of me; I regretted my words. Niko was a kid, not quite sixteen, a good kid brought up in a different world to mine. I said 'sorry'.

He stared at the ground, slowly shaking his head. 'Don't worry, you just don't get it, that's all. My epilepsy, it's different, that gay stuff, it's just …' He paused, desperate to find the right words. 'It's just so wrong. I saw two guys kissing in McDonald's the other day. It made me want to vomit.'

'What would you do if one of your children was gay? Would you hate them?' He said this would never happen to a child of his.

'It could happen to anyone. You probably even know someone who is gay, but don't realise it.'

'None of my friends are gay and my friends know I'm not gay.' He spoke with absolute conviction. 'When I was thirteen my friends bought me a woman to prove I was not gay.'

Surely he hadn't said what I thought he'd just said.

'You had sex with a prostitute when you were thirteen years old?'

He shrugged his shoulders. 'It's normal; all my friends did the same thing.'

Was this a reflection of a small group of friends, or an established part of growing up where he had? It didn't matter. Here I was trying to tell this individual to not hate gays, and to give up vodka, when I was clueless about him and the world he lived in.

'We're not here to talk about this, but about you and your medication.'

Niko claimed he had simply forgotten to pick up his tablets, and denied planning a drinking binge. 'I'm not stupid. I know the risks.' I chose to trust him, but warned him that I would be checking on him every day to make sure he had taken them.

So much of my job seems to be helping people to co-exist, despite themselves. But nobody is actually born to hate. The biggest influences in deciding whom you like or dislike are your parents, followed by your friends and, of course, the society you live in. I've met gay Iranians, Egyptians, Russians, Kazaks, Americans, Brazilians; the list goes on.

Aside from the normal gripes every employee has with their

employer, our school has little bullying, violence is rare, and kids from all walks of life love it here, because they really are accepted and can fit in.

The lesson for me is learning not to judge those who have opinions I disagree with, because if I did that then I'd never be able even to talk to someone like Niko. You are who you are and, I truly believe, meaningful change has to come from within. I just hope Nico, and many other young people like him, find that change in their lifetimes.

Celine

As well as offering a friendly ear and advice, my role is to support the specialist counsellor at the school tackle the big issues. Unfortunately, staff don't always see eye to eye.

You can't counsel someone with bulimia without monitoring other possible symptoms. And you can't offer sound medical treatment without knowing all the facts. If I don't know a patient is bulimic, as one counsellor chose to keep from me, I can't do my job.

I kept seeing the one poor girl because of stomach pains and burning sensations in her chest. I ended up referring her to Dr Fritz, who passed her on to a gastroenterologist. She was about to have an endoscopy – a procedure that passes a camera into the stomach – when the counsellor finally told me what was wrong. The counsellor felt she was betraying her patient because she was the first person they'd confided in.

There's a fine balance between keeping confidentiality and informing those who need to know. Fortunately our next counsellor, Cathy, had too much common sense to hold onto such secrets. Cathy had spent time as a psychologist working in a psychiatric ward before becoming a school counsellor. She oozed experience. And we'd need all the help we could get …

*

'There's blood everywhere, you have to come now, she's cut her wrists, I'm calling an ambulance,' screeched Lisa. I told her to apply pressure before I hung up the phone and dashed to the car, hurling my medical kit in the back.

They say 'one in ten' people will self-harm at some point in their life, but it often feels like so many more. You begin to wonder if it's a normal part of growing up, but I think it seems that way because it only takes one victim to draw you into their circle of pain and torment. The signs are not always glaringly obvious, but the effects can last a lifetime.

At two o'clock on a Monday morning I received a call about Celine, a fourteen-year-old girl from Canada. Celine had decided to play with a razor. Her wrists weren't cut in the traditional manner (across the wrist) or even the more effective manner (longitudinally along the length of the artery), instead she had cut out a rectangular section of skin about 1mm in depth by about 4cm by 2cm on both her wrists. The edges weren't ragged, but cut with clean strokes. There was plenty of blood, but no damage to the veins, or the arteries, that I could see.

It was just as well no vessels were cut as she'd waited two hours before deciding to get help from her friend Lisa, during which time she probably would have died if she had severed something important.

'Why'd you do it?' I asked as I placed a dressing on her arm. The middle of a crisis is not the best time to psychoanalyse, but I also needed to make conversation, to keep my patient involved in what was going on. Sometimes girls shrink into themselves, and don't say a thing. This worries me more than the ones who talk, even if it is just superficial. Having the energy to engage in your surroundings and the people around you is a good sign.

'It makes me feel better.' As far as I can tell, this seems to be true in self-harm cases. Generally, no matter what the cause, whether it is sadness, anger, self-loathing, guilt, or a combination of them all, the actual cutting seems to temporarily relieve the sufferer from their worries. The physical pain helps relieve the mental agony. Celine was content to let me dress her wound, but when I suggested that I should take her to hospital, she began to resist.

'It's not a big deal,' she said, as if this was an everyday occurrence. 'I won't do it again.' I asked if this was her first time, and she said it was. I had to be sure, but it didn't seem that now was the time to push, so I went into the hall, leaving Celine with Lisa, while I called Cathy down.

'Is she one of yours?' I asked when Cathy arrived. She nodded. But before she got a chance to explain, Lisa called out.

'She's trying to take off the dressing. You have to stop her.'

Cathy and I hurried inside.

'I just wanted to see it again; see how bad it is. I'm sorry,' she said, her voice cracking. I went outside to call the ambulance while Cathy stayed with her. 'I'll go with you to hospital, you won't be alone.' Cathy was true to her word and stayed with Celine until she was admitted to a ward.

It wasn't until she got back that I found out a bit more of Celine's history.

'They found lots of scars on her upper thighs and hips.' Cathy was distraught, which was unusual for her because she had seen a lot of disturbing things in her time. 'It's been going on for some time.'

I realised then that Cathy was feeling guilty because she saw Celine once a month on a routine basis.

Cathy had a compulsory support group for the younger female students, the purpose of which was to stop minor issues before they became bigger problems, a sort of 'prophylactic' therapy. 'We even talked about self-harm a few weeks ago,' Cathy kept repeating.

Along with self-harm, the group discussed boys, schoolwork, study habits, dealing with stress, sleep habits and healthy eating.

'I can't believe I didn't see it.'

I'm sure Celine had no wish to kill herself, and while there is a good chance she will grow out of this and lead a normal life, the scars will remain forever, a permanent reminder.

With the help of the school and its staff, Celine stayed with us until graduation. She did not make any further attempts at hurting herself that we knew of.

'How can one person be so draining?' Cathy once asked after spending most of the night with Celine during a particularly bad time. They both knew that any further attempts would mean expulsion from school. Cathy and I both knew that it only takes one self-harmer to take up all your time, resources and energy – but there's no other way.

Such words may sound harsh, especially with the threat of expulsion; I have to give credit to our school for working hard to keep Celine. Many places have a zero tolerance towards such behaviour. It's not just a matter of taking up so much of everyone's time, there's a fear nestled in the back of any headmaster's mind, a little voice that asks 'what if …'

Girlfriend woes

Fortunately not all problems are as complicated or frightening as Celine's, but when you've got the perfect storm of teenagers, alcohol and hormones mixed up altogether, something – anything – could happen …

When you haven't got one, all you want to do is get one; when you've got one, everyone else's seems hotter than normal; and once you've actually managed the task of finding a suitable partner, strange things happen, it's almost as if a magnetic force is created that draws single women to you, and for the first time in your life you're desirable – but attached. These laws of attraction are a source of so much trouble.

At sixteen years of age Marcek was a handsome blend of Kiwi and Polish ancestry. 'The doctor said it was a good thing my dad married a Pole,' he told me once, 'because the gene pool in New Zealand is a bit limited.' Strange, but that was the same thing my doctor said when he found out I was married to a Polish woman.

It was because of this international connection that I got to know Marcek's family, and hence why I got to know Marcek better than most of the students at school.

He was softly spoken, I never heard him raise his voice or argue with a teacher, and the few times I saw him in the health centre were when he was genuinely ill. He didn't seem like someone who would do something rash or fall victim to the things a lot of young men do, but something happened one fateful Saturday night, and he snapped.

Marcek came to see me in my office on Monday morning, the knuckles on his right hand swollen and bruised. I suspected a case of GDGAPW syndrome: aka Get Drunk, Get Angry, Punch Wall. Sometimes the wall is substituted for a window or a person.

'What was it, a wall or face?'

'Huh?' He paused while thinking of a way out. 'It was the punching bag. I went too hard.'

As he didn't have any other signs of a fight, it was probably a wall.

'The wall will always win,' I said as I placed some ice on his swollen hand, but he stuck to his story. I would need to continue my investigation. I asked if he got up to much on Saturday night.

'Just a party. Was OK, I guess.' This was not the Marcek I knew, evasive and dishonest, and although I didn't want to know anything about the party, I did want to find out the truth. I could choose to ignore the real reason for his injury, request an x-ray and get the appropriate treatment, but what would he hit next time? The force he'd obviously used to punch whatever it was he had struck had been enough to probably break at least one bone in his hand, and next time the consequences could be much worse, for himself and for others.

'You have much to drink?'

'A bit.'

'How'd your girlfriend like the party?' I asked casually. 'What's her name again?'

Marcek swore under his breath in Polish. I reminded him I understood exactly what he'd just said.

'How the hell do you find out these things? Are there no secrets in this place?' Of course there are no secrets at a boarding school. We live and breathe gossip in this place, it's our lifeblood.

'Just tell me the truth about your hand, and then we'll go and get you an x-ray.'

I would never be so pushy with a patient in hospital, as they might just push back, but young men are masters of doing silly things, things that seem harmless but have serious consequences. If I was wrong and he'd hit someone's face, then the small laceration to his knuckle was much more serious because a tooth bite combined with a fracture around the knuckles is liable to get infected, and if not treated properly could cause permanent damage, and I told him so.

I also told him the story of an upcoming rugby star back in New Zealand who had punched a window. He cut some nerves in his right arm, and had to give up on possibly becoming an international rugby star. The sensation to his hand never fully returned and he had big problems catching the ball. 'The poor guy had to start playing soccer,' I explained.

'It's football, not soccer,' Marcek cut in, his mood seeming to lift. He seemed ready to talk.

'Let me guess, girlfriend trouble?'

'This is just wrong.' Marcek was shaking his head in disbelief. 'You're like a bloody detective. Anyone would think you're the party police.'

I'm not the party police, but I have become adept at filtering out the truth.

'We broke up, over nothing—' I cut him off, telling him I didn't need the details, I just wanted to know what he punched. 'I punched the wall. I was just drunk that's all. It's not a big deal.'

Marcek's x-ray showed a boxer's fracture. This sort of fracture happens when a regular Joe lashes out and doesn't punch correctly. A correctly thrown punch should connect with the second and third knuckles, but many people connect with the fourth and fifth (the ring and small finger) and one or both of them snap.

I convinced Marcek to have at least one meeting with the school counsellor to talk about dealing with anger; hopefully this was just a one-off, but when there is alcohol combined with women, anything is possible.

After my work was done, I thanked Marcek for his honesty, and told him I was sorry about the breakup.

'Oh, don't worry, we're back together. She thought I was paying too much attention to some girls, but I told her I wouldn't do that. We're good now, just the alcohol I guess.'

Fortunately fights within the school are not common, and people really do get along, with little bullying, and I'd go so far as to say that I'd feel happy letting my own children study here, which says it all. I think it's because everyone is often well travelled, or live in parts of the world where they might be in the minority – somehow this exposure makes them more tolerant of others, it's also because they don't have a choice but to get on, especially in such a small community. Children can't be responsible for the stupidity of their leaders, but they can be the future peacemakers and bringers of hope.

Right now with Russian and Ukrainian relations at such a low, the Russians and Ukrainians get along here. Violence does happen, but the worst cases I've seen or heard about have occurred when our children are outside the school.

Such as revenge beatings: one poor eighteen-year-old lad had crossed a couple of Serbians, and during a weekend trip to a nearby city, was set upon by a group of Serbs who weren't part of the school.

Another time, a group of students had a run in with some Eastern Europeans who were rumoured to have a diamond smuggling operation. One of the 'mafia' lads waved a gun around, and although this turned out to be a fake, it scared a lot of people, and ended up in a police investigation, which turned up nothing. More recently, some of the boys from a visiting French football team took a particular fancy to some of our schoolgirls and became a bit pushy. The students rallied to the defence of their women and one of our students received a bottle to the head in return.

These outside events usually take place when the students have been excused from school by their parents. Do these parents have any idea what their children get up to? Of course not – even the well-meaning ones often don't have a clue, they probably prefer it that way.

CHAPTER SEVEN

In Loco Parentis

Naif

I try my best, but I can't help wonder about the parents whose children I'm in charge of, and I can't help comparing my own actions as a parent myself, and the actions of my own mum and dad as well.

I don't know how I compared to Naif's parents (he certainly never talked about them) but naturally I developed an idea of who I imagined them to be. It was clear Naif's relationship with his father wasn't ideal.

It's sad that some children don't get along with their fathers. Of course, sometimes it's justified, but often hormones and the nature of teenage life play a part too. I hoped Naif didn't hate his father, after all, he'd spent a lot of money making sure his son got the best schooling money can buy. Surely that must mean he cares?

Unfortunately, generosity doesn't always equate to interest.

'I need their permission to give you the shot.' I was harassing Naif, trying to get him to give me a valid email or phone number, because he required a tetanus shot, and I needed written consent, but his parents weren't responding. The tetanus shot wasn't vital, but he'd cut his hand in art class and according to his records it looked like he had missed this routine childhood vaccination.

'They're busy people; you won't get a reply,' he explained. 'I'm old enough to look after myself. You don't need their permission. I'm eighteen anyway.' I suspected Naif was very capable of looking after himself. He had a confident, street savvy wariness about him. He was smooth, but not in an arrogant youthful way – more like the characters from the movie *Goodfellas*. Naif had the greased hair, the fine clothes; he looked like a clichéd mobster, even when just going to class! School rules didn't apply to him apparently; he had his own dress code, his own flashy style.

I reassured his ego that 'of course' he could look after himself and that I only needed written consent because those were the rules.

'Just give me the number in your phone, and I'll talk to them.' All families give the school the usual contact numbers, such as home and mobile, but a lot of kids also have a private line to yet another phone, a line that they can always contact their parents on. I've used this line a number of times when unable to contact a parent on the regular phone numbers they give us.

'There's no need to call them, they'll get in touch, just give it a break. Don't call them again, all right?' He was trying to sound casual, as if he was doing me a favour, but why was he so sensitive? Why wouldn't his parents respond to my calls and emails?

'Let's forget the tetanus for now,' I said, sensing tension. It wasn't urgent. Even the local hospitals have stopped giving the shot, as most of them have never seen a case. 'But for future reference, I do need to be able to speak to your father. What if there's an emergency?'

'You don't understand, sir. I've been looking after myself for a long time. I live my own life. I don't need my father. I don't want a father. You don't need to speak to my father, ever.' Naif was suddenly conscious of the words that had escaped against his will and began to retreat.

'Just forget, it all right?' he said, as he stormed out the room. With his usual panache, of course.

I first met Naif when he was only fourteen years old. His first words to me had been to complain about the temperature:

'It's so cold here, this is ridiculous.' Naif was from somewhere in the Middle East and this was his first winter on a mountain.

'It's too cold for school, sir. Let me rest in the health centre. I'll make it worth your while.' Naif had pulled out his wallet and begun rifling through a thick wad of notes. I took the wallet and told him to go to class. 'It doesn't work like that.'

'It's not fair,' he protested as I guided him back out the door and handed his wallet back to him.

Many kids 'pretend' to bribe me so they can miss class and go back to bed, although I have the funny suspicion that if I really did take the money, they'd be fine with it.

But other than the fact that Naif always had a wallet full of cash, I knew nothing of his background. Our interactions were frequent but usually brief, pleasant but superficial. He would poke his head through the door every so often, to ask how I was, complain about the cold, or ask if there was a bed free. The answers were nearly always the same, 'I'm fine', 'It's not that cold', followed by 'No – now go to class.'

Naif didn't return the next school year, as well as the one after that. I had forgotten all about him when he came back to finish his senior year of high school.

'Do you remember me? Surely you can't have forgotten me,' Naif quipped, as if the previous two years' absence were nothing. I hadn't forgotten him; I just didn't recognise him.

'What happened to your face?' Perhaps it wasn't the welcome back he was hoping for, but he had changed in ways that didn't seem regular adolescent growth could account for. 'Broke my nose,' he explained. It wasn't just his nose. Naif was pale and had lost a lot of weight. Naif had never been fat, but he hadn't filled out at all, his face looked gaunt and he looked frail.

Naif visited me and the other nurses regularly, he continued to try and buy his way into a bed, all the while flattering us and always taking an interest. But there was something different about him that I couldn't quite explain; a seriousness that wasn't there before. He mingled with his peers, but didn't participate fully in the usual parties or some of the more silly antics that senior kids usually get up to, although he still flashed plenty of cash.

His biggest expense that term was paying the bill for the champagne shower he and his friends had participated in at a nightclub one Saturday night. The boys had clocked up 35,000 euros on bubbly they hadn't even drunk, but shaken and sprayed on boys from another boarding school. At least three schools had been involved and each had similar bills.

As usual, Naif couldn't figure out how I found out about the party. On this occasion, the fools had posted a copy of the bill to Facebook and it had eventually made its way to the headmaster's office. They'd been competing to see which school could generate the most expensive bill.

I'd raised the story more as a matter of interest. They hadn't done anything wrong; they were of age and had been checked out with their 'parents' for the weekend, but I did remind Naif that he shouldn't drink so much.

'I don't drink, sir,' he declared, his tone serious. Naif denied touching a drop. 'I only sprayed it around. I don't drink.' I told him he wasn't a good liar and he vehemently denied he had been drinking. 'I may lie about some stuff, but not about that.'

Maybe he was telling the truth.

A couple of weeks later Naif and I were at the local doctor's office because he was suffering from a nasty throat infection and was going to need antibiotics. He was coughing so much I expected to see a bit of lung come up. When the doctor asked him if he had any previous health problems, Naif replied:

'I had pancreatitis about a year ago.'

Dr Fritz didn't believe what he heard, and neither did I. He asked Naif to repeat what he had just said, and Naif confirmed he definitely had pancreatitis. Was that why he had left school so abruptly? He hadn't seemed sick at the time.

Pancreatitis is rare in someone so young. It's a life threatening illness and there is no cure. They put you on a drip, keep you nil by mouth, stick a tube up your nose and into your stomach to empty it out, monitor your blood sugars, and give you massive doses of morphine and antibiotics, for days or even weeks. It's not unusual to end up in intensive care. The treatment revolves around giving your body absolute rest and to be pain free, while you hope for the best.

'Are you sure it's pancreatitis you're thinking of?' I asked. 'It's a very serious problem. I've never heard of someone as young as you getting it.'

'Well, I can never drink alcohol again or I could die, so I know how serious it is.' Pancreatitis is a problem usually associated with alcoholics.

Naif then told me the rest of the story …

When he had suddenly left school at the age of fourteen, he had moved to London to study. His father had put him up in an apartment, and left him alone with a family friend.

'He's our driver,' Naif explained when I asked who the family friend was, but he sounded much more as if he was a roommate, bought his alcohol for him, and doubled as a bodyguard.

'I always have a bodyguard,' Naif admitted, 'except when I come here. It's safe here.'

Instead of studying or going to school, Naif became a teenage alcoholic. The only adults in his life were his 'driver' and the women he bought.

'You wouldn't believe the world I live in,' Naif said, and to demonstrate he flicked through at random some pictures from his iPhone. There were images of cars, nightclubs and women; very gorgeous women and a very sophisticated looking young man. The clothes and shades may have convinced others he was a wealthy man, but all I saw was a rich, lost boy.

After surviving his close call with pancreatitis Naif had spent twelve weeks in an alcohol rehabilitation centre for young people. He claims it has worked, but knowing that you could die the next time you drink is a pretty good incentive for staying sober.

Naif graduated from high school. He stayed off the alcohol, doesn't take drugs, is in university, although the money hasn't dried up. He posts pictures on Facebook of him driving his Ferrari, or sunbathing on some foreign beach. In all the photos I see of him, he still looks a sickly and pale young man, although a very well-dressed one.

I never once heard him talk about his parents, and have yet to even see a picture of them … although it's probably best I never met them, as who knows what I would have said or done.

David

While it is often hard getting in touch with parents, it's usually for a benign reason: they're on a plane or in an undeveloped place that is rich in oil and minerals but lacking in modern technology. Often these circumstances result in children that have learnt to fend for themselves.

David was a good regular. By 'good regular' I mean he didn't come to the health centre to avoid class. He was rarely sick. Instead, he liked to come and talk to us during lunch break because, in his eyes, we were the only people he could talk to normally. He had an air of maturity that only a handful of eighteen-year-olds do.

'I can't talk to anyone else around here. They're just bloody stupid.' Normally, I'd suggest that David's remark was unfair, but he probably had a good point. He didn't join in the usual hijinks that other boys got up to.

'Mate, I've done it all before. It's all I've done since I was fourteen. I'm tired of that shit.' This was no kid before me, but an old soul in a teenager's body.

I knew very little of David's background, except that he had joined the school for his senior year of high school. As I've mentioned earlier, it's unusual for students to enrol for their final year, and I was naturally curious.

'Why did you leave England?' I asked. David shrugged his shoulders. 'Too strict.'

'What about that school in the States you were enrolled at? Why'd you leave that one?'

'Just got bored.'

'Why'd you come here?'

'The snow; and I hear it's pretty relaxed.'

David knew boarding schools better than anyone I'd ever met. Since the age of eight he'd spent his life in and out of various schools in Britain, America, Africa and Europe.

'So where's home?' I asked and he couldn't give me a straight answer. He couldn't actually identify a place which he called home. His accent wasn't quite American or British, and although English was his first language, he was fluent in French, Spanish, German and rapidly grasping the fundamentals of Russian.

'You've been around a bit. What do your parents think of all this?'

'They don't mind, as long as I graduate.' The supposed attitude of indifference of his parents matched David's own.

'You sound like an old man before your time.' David just grinned.

'They let me do what I like, as long as my grades are good, and I stay out of trouble, and don't do drugs. They said if I graduate high school they'll pay for me to spend a year anywhere I like.'

David planned to spend six months travelling around South America, and the other six months seeing Vietnam, Thailand and Cambodia. I also found out that he had spent the last summer break travelling with friends in a van around Europe.

When I was his age there was no way I'd have the know-how or confidence to do what he had just done, and no way my parents would have let me even if we had the money, and I told him so. 'Yeah, well, I've had to raise myself. I don't see much of my folks.'

Between the ages of eight and thirteen, David spent on average two months a year with his parents. If he wasn't in boarding school, he was in summer school, and when he was older, he began to develop a circle of friends in similar situations. They would spend their vacation time at each other's holiday homes, and by the time they were sixteen, they began exploring independently.

David loved his parents and, at least on the surface, seemed happy with his life. I was also impressed by how mature he was, and by what he'd accomplished in such a short time. Yet, I felt sorry for David, even though I have no right to. I suppose it's just natural to assume that the way you were raised was healthier than others who are different. All the same, I could never imagine being an absent parent. I love seeing my children too much. And isn't that what being a parent is all about?

Edward

Unlike David, Edward had a home. It was here, with us. He'd been here five years.

He was the perfect student: handsome, polite, good at school, he didn't smoke or do drugs (well, he'd passed every drug test!) and he was popular with his peers. He wasn't abandoned here; his parents visited regularly and he spent every break with them. I liked his parents and I wanted to emulate their success. If my kids turn out like Edward, I'll be happy.

But how well did I know Edward? Five years is a long time, you begin to think you know all there is to know about a person, but then they surprise you. I did know that Edward appreciated what he had; the chance of a good education, in a safe environment, while still being able to follow his passion. Edward was good at sports, especially football, and if his grades continued the way they had last year, he had a good chance of finishing his senior year in the top three of the school. As an active boy with the right attitude, I wouldn't normally have come to know Edward at all as he rarely visited the health centre. But Edward's passion for skiing nearly rivalled my own.

'You've got a sweet life,' Edward said to me. It was a quiet Friday afternoon and we were watching a clip on my work computer of some extreme skiing. Friday afternoons used to be very busy, but since management (very cleverly) made a rule that if you are sick on a Friday, then you don't get to go out Friday night, things changed.

I do have a good quality of life, I can't deny that. Living in a small mountain town in a developed nation has its advantages. It's clean, you're constantly walking either uphill or down so you're always exercising, and the crime is negligible. The local police officer usually turns his bedroom light off at ten, so if you are going to do something nefarious, you know the best time to begin. But then the police won't have difficulty trying to find you as everyone knows who you are and where you live. I started to feel uncomfortable with Edward's description of my life. 'I don't just sit around watching YouTube all day,' I replied defensively. 'I had to work to get to this stage,' I added.

Edward gave a brief chuckle then explained exactly what he meant. 'I mean you live in a ski town and go up the mountain whenever you want; and when you're not skiing, you only have to look after a bunch of spoilt kids.'

'You're being a bit hard, aren't you? They're not all spoilt. They didn't choose their parents.'

'Perhaps, but I'm not like them. Don't make that mistake.' I promised I wouldn't.

'The job isn't always easy. You've been here long enough to know what winters are like. Sickness, ski injuries, broken bones. It's a nightmare.'

'Yeah man, but c'mon, what more do you need out of life than to ride? You're living the dream, even when you're old.' He actually meant what he said, about my age that is.

I once felt the same way, but there was no need to tell Edward how that changes for most people. Growing up and having a family changes everything, usually for the better, and he would either find that out for himself, or not. If that's his dream, I'm not going to deter him, although I did ask one favour of him.

'Please promise me before becoming a ski bum, you finish university.'

'Don't think I have much choice.'

'Good,' I added, my tone brisk, not asking for an explanation.

While Edward would soon be a young adult, like most people his age a bit of direction from family is a good thing. My parents had said exactly the same thing to me: 'Make sure you get an education, and then you can ski.'

During ski season, the first sign of a problem is often in the grades. Edward's tan deepened as his grades dropped.

'They'll pick up,' he said to me one day on the chairlift. When I commented that he didn't seem worried he said his parents were more worried than him.

'Dad went to Princeton, so he expects me to do the same.'

'You won't get accepted to Princeton with average grades,' I said, and the conversation died briefly as he paused, as if unsure what to say.

'Who said I want to go to Princeton?' he blurted out. I kept silent.

'I'd prefer Colorado anyway.' Colorado is great for skiing, and if I were in his place, I'd choose the same, as it would mean a university education as well as endless powder skiing on my doorstep.

By February Edward's grades had dropped even further; he was barely passing his Maths class. His tan was still beaming, but he wasn't the same. He wouldn't come and talk with me like he used to and he had even begun to miss some of his classes. Rumour had it he'd taken up smoking, and he'd been in a fight with his roommate. I only heard about these things through the people dealing with his discipline issues, but soon

I was involved far more than I wanted to be.

In late March I received a call from a teacher in Edward's dorm. 'I think he's taken something, he won't stay awake.' There are some words that always make your skin crawl and your stomach sink, as well as make you run.

'Call the ambulance. I'm on my way.'

Edward wasn't unconscious when I got there. He was sitting on the floor, his head in the toilet, vomit dribbling down his chin. He was mumbling a phrase, over and over. I crouched beside him, placing my arm across his shoulders, straining to hear what he was saying. 'I'm sorry, so sorry.'

'What happened?'

'I'm so sorry, so sorry,' he said again, turning his head towards me.

'His roommate called me and said he thinks he's taken something,' explained Mr Fisher, the teacher on duty that evening. 'I ran here and called you straight away.'

'What have you taken?' I asked.

'Just some Tylenol. I'm sorry.'

Tylenol, an American brand of paracetamol, is one of the worst drugs to overdose on but is often the most common. Perhaps because it's accessible over the counter, people think it's harmless. In correct dosages it is safe, but too much, even a small overdose and it can damage the liver severely. There is an antidote, and so the sooner Edward was taken to hospital the better.

Mr Fisher confirmed that he had called the ambulance, but it was forty minutes away. I briefly contemplated taking Edward to hospital myself as I didn't want to waste so much time, but decided against it. If he started vomiting again, lost consciousness or any of the dozen other things that could go wrong happened, I wouldn't be able to do a thing. He could die in transit.

Edward wasn't able to give us a clear idea of how many pills he'd taken, although there was a half-empty bottle of vodka. His roommate confirmed that he had seen this bottle the day before and it had been full.

Edward was taken to hospital by ambulance and I spent the next twelve hours at his bedside.

This story does have a happy ending. Although Edward had taken twenty or so tablets, fortunately he had vomited most of them up almost as soon as he'd taken them. While his blood tests showed only a mildly elevated level of paracetamol, he was commenced on the antidote, and his liver function tests ended up being fine.

Naturally I wanted to ask him why? But I was hesitant. The acute stage of an illness is not always the best time to delve in to find meaningful answers. The physical needs must come first, and when you ask these questions you ask yourself if you're asking because you want to help, or because you're desperate for an explanation. You want to know if there was something you could have done to prevent it. Yet sometimes asking questions at this time, when they're the most vulnerable, is when you can get the most honest answer.

I managed to stave off my curiosity until the following morning, twelve hours later, when he was sober and rested.

'I never wanted to go to Princeton,' he explained. 'But my father will disown me if I don't go.' I told him he must have been exaggerating.

'You don't know my father. He offered to buy me a Lamborghini if I got in. I guess I won't be getting one now.' I asked him what he wanted to do.

'My father wants me to be a lawyer. I don't know what I want. I don't want to be a lawyer though.'

I had very little contact with Edward's parents during this ordeal as this was done through the headmaster, but during the ten minutes I did spend talking with Edward's father, I could hear the worry, the fear, and the utter heartache coming through loud and clear. Edward broke into tears when I told him this.

Edward is now a grown man. He wasn't disowned. He spent two winters living his dream working in a ski resort and eventually got his ski instructor's licence.

He did end up going to college, but graduated as a PE teacher, not a lawyer. He works at a boarding school that has a large focus on winter sports and he is one of the coaches of the ski team. He learned that his parents only wanted the best for him, and for him to be happy. It turns out they had no idea their son didn't want what they wanted.

Edward's story made me realise the immense pressure many of my students have upon them. My parents always wanted me to do well, but I never felt forced to follow a path they chose for me. I now have a greater appreciation of the expectations some of the children have. As it turns out, I'm just glad Edward found his way, is happy, and is currently living his own dream.

Rich personalities

When Franco was asked to leave school he slipped away quietly, which was unusual for him because he was a flashy, seventeen-year-old fiery Italian. He talked a lot and dressed in ways that in many places would have got him beaten up.

'You know nothing,' he told me when I suggested that his choice of clothes wasn't the most appropriate for the winter weather.

'We don't all dress like we're from a farm.' I had discovered him in the hallway about to head into a blizzard with only a shirt, a sleeveless vest, and dress shoes.

Franco had a talent for putting together irritating combinations of words that made me rise to the bait. I've heard much worse, but it wasn't what he'd said, it was the arrogance behind the words. I never once spoke to my teachers in such a manner, it would have been a sure way to get detention or, depending on the teacher, a caning. Manners need to be taught and sometimes enforced. As I marched him back to the health centre for a piece of my mind, I zipped up my fleece, hiding my plaid shirt.

'I'll be late for class,' he protested.

Franco had around $10,000 worth of clothes on, excluding his watch, and for all the money spent, he still didn't have solid shoes for the snow, or a proper jacket to combat the cold. If he wanted to slip on the ice and freeze to death, then that was fine with me, but I was not going to let him get away with talking to me in such a tone.

'Listen *mate*, I may know "nothing" of fashion, but I do know how to talk to people.'

Franco tried to back-pedal, the arrogance gone. 'Hey, I didn't mean it in a bad way, it's just you know …' He left the thought hanging as he realised he was probably going to make matters worse, but I told him to go on.

'Well, we're sophisticated over here, we know style. In Italy we wear only the best. You're from a country of farmers; it's not your fault, nothing personal.'

The cocksure little brat actually believed what he said, but then maybe he was right.

I have to confess that I did struggle with Franco's handbag. 'It's Louis Vuitton, made just for men,' he explained, rolling his eyes. I thought they made things to do with sailing, all New Zealanders knew that, the discovery they made man-bags was disturbing. I asked what the eagle symbol on his belt buckle meant and discovered it was worth over $2,000. 'It's crocodile skin,' he said casually. I had to substantially revise my estimation upwards of his outfit's value.

Perhaps if Franco paid as much attention to school life as he did to how he looked, he might not have been asked to leave, but school wasn't important to him. All that mattered was looking good, especially for the ladies.

Franco finally apologised to me, and he sounded genuinely sorry. I wondered if I'd been a little harsh. Perhaps I'd only imagined the arrogance in his voice; maybe I was the one with the chip on the shoulder. My 'giving him a piece of my mind' had turned into an education and self-reflection session for both of us.

Franco never wore $10 trousers or $5 t-shirts – he wouldn't be seen dead in such things. 'You have to look good for the ladies … all the time,' he explained.

'But don't you want a woman to like you for who you are?' I asked. Franco found this genuinely puzzling.

'Women are interested in what you wear, how nice you look, how good you smell and the car you drive.' Franco usually had girls hanging around him. He was a very handsome lad, but other than his money, this seemed the only other thing he had going for him.

In an ideal world, this meeting would be the perfect opportunity to show him how wrong he was, to discuss meaningful relationships, and how being your true self is what is important. I could have explained how a good woman wants to see the real Franco. But I could be wrong.

Franco's world is full of glitz and glamour, from supercars to supermodels. His father has been on the cover of magazines, his mother makes the headlines dating politicians, rock stars and billionaires. Perhaps Franco is right, at least in his circle of friends.

'You've seen my latest.' It was a statement, not a question. There was no way anyone could not notice his latest girlfriend, a Brazilian student, with whom he would walk to and from every class latched to her arm, making out with her outside of, during, and after class. She was attractive and older, but surely this relationship would end up just like the rest – another conquest.

'Of course,' I said.

'You gotta know how to please your woman,' he added.

I'd had enough. I wasn't going to be told how to please a woman by a seventeen-year-old boy. All I'd wanted to do was make him change his shoes so he didn't slip on the ice, or catch pneumonia because looking cool was better than staying warm, and now we were talking about women, fashion, comparing his world to mine.

He finally agreed to change into some proper winter clothes after I threatened him with detention.

Franco never graduated from school. He never really even bothered to turn up to class. It's unusual for someone to be asked to leave for failing grades, but when you not only skip class, but leave the village without permission, it's a basic safety issue. The school needs to know where you are at all times, and as the school couldn't keep track of him, he was deemed a safety risk. 'Dad thinks I should be in school. I'm just here to keep him happy,' Franco told me one day when I asked him why he wasn't even trying. When I asked him what he was going to do instead, he just shrugged his shoulders and said, 'Enjoy life … enjoy the women.'

A few days after Franco had been 'withdrawn' from the school, the headmaster came to me and handed me an object the cleaners had found in his room. It's not unusual for the cleaning staff to find unusual objects or strange substances, from heroin to blow-up dolls, but Franco had something that had me bewildered, a small tube of gel, with various chemical ingredients.

The moment I got a hit from Google I warned Mr Driscoll not to touch it again. 'Get if off my desk,' I said, handing him some rubber gloves.

'I'm not touching it! You get rid of it,' demanded a suddenly worried headmaster. 'What the hell is it?'

'It's lignocaine,' I began, but the name meant nothing to him and I told him it's a common anaesthetic. 'Though it's not commonly used as a penis-desensitiser.' Mr Driscoll grabbed the alcohol hand wash from my desk and applied liberally.

'Damn him,' I thought. Franco had had the last laugh.

Expulsion

Franco wasn't the first student I knew to be expelled. Although, it's not really called that. They say 'withdrawn' instead. Maybe this makes the parents feel better, but for those in the education business, it's code for 'something bad happened but we won't tell you what it is'. Schools don't like to tell other schools what the 'bad' thing was, they believe in giving everyone a fresh start. It's pretty fair, and unless you break specific rules, it's surprisingly hard to be kicked out of school. I think it's because, according to Mr Driscoll, 'there's no such thing as a bad child, just bad behaviour'. If any of you reading want to get withdrawn from my school, you will need to break one (or more) of the following:

Drugs

Any drug will do, except for alcohol and cigarettes. Part of my role involves drug testing and education, and cannabis through to heroin will see you instantly expelled. Depending on the country, if a drug test is positive, the school informs the family and advises them to leave the country, as they are legally bound to inform the police, who have to prosecute.

Cigarettes

Expulsion is an option for repeat offenders, but considering that 30 per cent of the students smoke, this is unlikely to be the sole reason for exclusion.

Alcohol

Again, only repeat offenders, and always tricky, especially with the Eastern Europeans as they use vodka for medicinal purposes. Vodka and black pepper apparently works for stomach upsets, and while we've confiscated bottles from rooms, students have avoided being reprimanded because their parents protested.

Stealing

Often instant expulsion, although the case has to be airtight. Rumours can be true, exaggerated or completely wrong, and a wrong accusation can damage an innocent person's reputation, even force them to change school. It's an intermittent problem and most of it seems more opportunistic than planned, such as a student leaving their wallet in the lounge, and someone taking it, rather than a concerted effort to break into a room or locker.

Spending the night in another dorm

This can go either way, although generally boys in girls' dorms means dismissal, but it also depends on age. Even with consent, it doesn't look good if parents hear there was a group of senior boys in a dorm of underage girls.

Sex

Realistically, if this carried an instant punishment, we'd be expelling half the school. And while the school rules say 'hand-holding' only, I've known Mr Driscoll to bump into students in action, and instead of stopping them himself, come and ask me to deal with it. I think he thinks that by having nothing to do with 'it' he can deny any responsibility.

Fighting

Again this depends on the seriousness of any injuries sustained, the reasons why, and whether it's a one-off or an on-going problem. Often groups of kids will occasionally clash based on cultures, the Saudi students and the Brazilians, or the Russian students and the Americans. They play on each other's stereotypes, and in the process live up to their own. But generally, and unlike most schools, fighting is not a problem.

Self-harm

Cutting and burning are the most common and lasting. Generally, this isn't grounds for expulsion, but forced withdrawal for health reasons, although it's not automatic. It depends on the counsellor's verdict and whether she thinks we can deal with the problem. A student may get one chance if they've cut only once while at school, but if they do so again, then they have to go. One self-harmer can take all of the counsellor's time and energy. It's often sad to see the students removed, as we're sometimes the only security they've had, but cutting spreads; I swear it almost becomes fashionable.

Unfortunately, we sometimes have to let students go, even when we really are the best place for them.

Maria

'Can I bring my daughter on the thirteenth?' asked Mr Ricardo.

Alana explained that school began on August twentieth.

'But I can pay. It's not a problem.'

Alana had spent the last three years working in admissions, and this was the first time someone had tried to drop off their child early. She again explained that it wasn't about paying someone to look after his daughter, but the fact that none of the staff would be on campus by that date.

'Are you absolutely sure?' For the third time Alana turned him down.

'What day is the twentieth then?'

Alana told him it was a Saturday.

The summer passed without incident and too quickly, as usual. The Friday night before opening day was the first cool evening of the season. Late summer in the mountains is unpredictable; the day is scorching hot, then you're greeted the next morning with a dusting of snow on the surrounding peaks. If you're new to the mountains it's easy to get caught out, especially if you go out for a drink and let the alcohol numb your senses.

Mike and Christie's senses weren't numb. They were boarding school veterans; they had spent a decade in the mountains, and never got caught out by the weather. They'd spent the evening at the local pub catching up with the returning staff. At 12.30am, they decided to call it a night and began the fifteen-minute walk home.

On their way home they had to walk past the girls' dormitory; an empty, old building, made depressingly creepy by the lack of life. But … there was life there that night. Next to the main door was the silhouette of a child. Surprised, Mike and Christie went to investigate.

They found a young, olive-skinned girl huddled against the wall, clutching her bag to her chest in an attempt to keep warm.

'Are you from the school?' she asked. Christie knelt down beside her and told her she was. 'Why's it locked?' the girl blurted, before suddenly becoming suspicious. 'How do I know you're from the school?'

Christie opened her handbag and handed the girl her school ID card.

Christie asked how she ended up out here in the middle of the night. 'Dad dropped me off at midnight,' she stammered, shivering from the cold. Christie took off her jacket and wrapped it around her. 'He said that's when you're supposed to be open.' Christie and Mike couldn't believe what they were hearing. 'Your dad just left you here?'

'It wasn't actually Dad, it was my driver. But my driver was only doing what Dad told him to do.'

The girl's name was Maria. She was fourteen years old and from Brazil. She was Mr Ricardo's daughter. He obviously couldn't get rid of his daughter soon enough, and had chosen to take Alana's words literally. As of the stroke of midnight on the twentieth, school was open for business.

What does one do with a child abandoned on the side of a mountain? You get them inside, give them something warm to drink, and call the headmaster.

Maria spent her first morning in the health centre catching up on some rest while Mr Driscoll tried to contact her parents.

It should have been a police matter, but since when has doing the right thing been so straightforward? A child who had just flown in from the other side of the world, abandoned on the side of the mountain, in the middle of the night. It took two days before someone from administration finally got hold of Mr Ricardo.

He was apologetic, but insisted it was a misunderstanding about when the school was to be open. He added that his driver had made a simple mistake, and promised to sort the situation out.

Fortunately, Maria didn't seem too shocked by the whole ordeal, and instead of 'resting' she was busy telling us and anyone who would listen about life back in Brazil: 'You don't want to piss off my dad.'

Michaela told Maria that the school had already been in contact with her father and that he had apologised about the misunderstanding.

'And you believed him?' asked an incredulous Maria. 'This was no mistake. My parents couldn't wait to get rid of me. They don't know what to do with me.'

The young, abandoned girl from Brazil was beginning to show some teeth.

'I'm sure your parents want you,' offered an uncertain sounding Michaela.

'Then why'd they dump me here? Why aren't they angry about the whole mess? I bet he blamed it on the driver. My driver isn't stupid. He always follows orders to the letter. But I don't care.'

I suspected she did care, otherwise she wouldn't have raised her voice and become so animated, so angry. That's what kids do when something is wrong at home. They pretend they don't care, but it's just a show – a shell to protect themselves.

Michaela changed tack and began to talk about all the good things that Maria had to look forward to at school. She also stressed to Maria that she was welcome to come and visit us in the health centre anytime, even if she wasn't sick.

Maria promised to take her up on her offer, although not without giving a warning first: 'You don't know what you've got yourselves into.' I hoped she was only joking.

Within a few weeks, problems had begun to arise. Cathy had met with Maria regularly, and kept us up to date on how she was doing. 'Things have been going missing in her dorm. But Maria insists she's innocent.'

The bottle of vodka the cleaning staff found in her room was the next complaint. Though it was unopened, she denied it was hers. Apparently she only drinks rum. Alcohol offences are taken seriously, even seniors with drinking permissions aren't allowed alcohol in their room. Given her age, she could have been expelled if it had been found opened.

As a result Maria began to spend more time being counselled by Cathy. All students who have alcohol infractions have to see the counsellor, usually as a 'one-off', but Maria was an exception.

'She's started smoking,' Cathy told us. 'She's the most cheerful lost child I've seen in a long time.' Like nurses, counsellors are bound by confidentiality but Cathy does tell us what we need to know. 'But I think if you scratch beneath the surface you'll find a whole lot of anger, and a very frightened little girl.'

It wasn't long before Maria got into her first fight; a hair-pulling contest between her and her now ex-roommate. The usual words were slung with ever increasing ferocity and decreasing creativity – 'you thief', 'you cow', 'you bitch', 'you fat bitch', 'you ho', 'you slag', and finally 'you slut'. Sadly 'thief' stuck and a search of Maria's wardrobe uncovered some shoes and a coat that belonged to the ex-roommate. Maria's defence was that her roommate had forgotten she'd lent them to her – a plausible story.

Meanwhile, the complaints were coming in thick and fast from teachers, dorm staff and parents.

If she continued on her path of self-destruction Maria would be sent home. The impact on the other students was simply too great, and we warned her of such. 'I'm never going home,' she insisted. 'Why would I ever want to? All Mum does is drink, and when Dad's not dragging her around the house by her hair, he's high on coke.'

If I had a dollar for every time a kid has lied, I'd have retired a very wealthy man years ago, but Maria's story felt different. It may have been the way she was dumped here, or the family that were impossible to contact, or her choice of words. She could have said that Dad 'beats Mum' but the words 'dragging Mum around the house by the hair' were very specific, too real for a young girl to make up? Perhaps.

Cathy said it was time to speak with the headmaster.

I suggested we go to the police, but Mr Driscoll said it was no use. 'It's the word of a wayward teenager against her family.' Isn't it always one person's word against another? I kept quiet, waiting for him to finish.

Cathy, Michaela and I asked Mr Driscoll if we should contact the child protection service, but he said that wouldn't help either.

'She's not an urgent case,' he explained, 'they're busy with urgent cases, with children in actual harm's way.'

This didn't feel right, but this isn't my home country. If a child made allegations like this in New Zealand, action would be swift.

'The moment the family hear anything suspicious, she'll be back in Brazil in the blink of an eye.'

If Maria was sent home, nothing would change, certainly not for the better. The school was the best place for her. It was for this reason that Mr Driscoll decided to keep her as long as we could. 'But she can't keep on being so disruptive, or I'll have no choice but to let her go.'

All schools have to make this decision at some stage; the future of the many versus the good of the one. Schools like ours have the added problem of being international. I don't know what laws there are in Saudi Arabia, Brazil, Iran, so we relied on Mr Driscoll's past experience in such matters.

Six months later, Maria was on her final warning. If she was caught smoking, stealing, fighting or missing another class, she'd be sent home. It was too late to change her failing grades to a pass, instead the challenge was to make it to class, and not be too disruptive.

The final straw came when Maria's parents gave their daughter permission to travel to a nearby city for the weekend, despite the fact she was not allowed to travel, according to school rules.

It's strange that when we want to contact a parent, it's often hard, but when the kids need permission to do something, they hound us until we accede to their wishes.

But what can you do when a 'family' member comes to pick them up?

So, one fateful Friday afternoon, Maria was driven away by her uncle who liked to dress as a chauffeur. Her uncle wasn't around when Maria drank herself unconscious; no parents, no aunts or cousins, not even the driver – an all too familiar scene. I was the one who the hospital contacted after finding her student identification in her purse, and I was the one who picked her up and took her back to school.

Maria made a full recovery, but her time was up. 'She's a danger to herself' was the general consensus. Even her father didn't put up a fight; he was probably already looking at the next school to send her to.

None of us heard from Maria again.

Enrolment by default

I'm not alone in thinking our school is the best place for some of our charges; some parents will go to extreme lengths to get their child enrolled in a good school.

Max was cool and stood out from the rest of the summer school kids. How does someone look cool? Well, true coolness doesn't come from trying; it's a confidence that comes from managing to survive life's ups and downs without being burned out or turning into an arsehole. In Max's case, this confidence made him appear older than his fifteen years, but in a good way. He was kind, helpful, said 'please' and 'thank you' and didn't argue. The image he presented was one that any parent would be proud of.

I first met Max during my one stint working with the summer school. Max spent the whole eight weeks of summer at school. Summer school is not really school, it's more like a summer camp run by different staff for a whole new set of kids; it's completely independent of the regular school. It's not unheard of for students to spend the whole eight weeks at summer school, but it doesn't tend to be a regular occurrence. I asked if Max normally spent his summer at camp.

'My parents are busy with the business,' he began to explain. His answer sounded rehearsed, the first sentence excusing his parents, his tone almost apologetic. 'But I've been to some awesome camps.' He proceeded to list the things he'd done over past summers: white water rafting, rock climbing, abseiling, bungee-jumping, paragliding … 'But I think this place is the best yet. My parents are going to enrol me for the school year.'

There's always a trickle of people from summer camp who end up enrolling for the regular school year, but Max was the exception. He didn't get accepted into the regular school year.

'It's bullshit' was how Max described the school's decision to exclude him. The decision surprised me as well, as most private schools are not always discerning when it comes to accepting students. Money talks, so there must be a big reason why he wasn't accepted. I asked him if he had any idea why they'd say no.

Max wasn't an idiot and didn't try to lie. 'Just some stuff,' he began, 'I did some stupid stuff in the past.' He wasn't going to elaborate and it was none of my business, but I wished him well, wherever he ended up.

Summer school came to an end and everyone went home, everyone except Max. No one could get hold of his parents or any relatives, and he had no flight booked home. The only contact the school received was through the accounts department, who had received three years' worth of tuition. That sort of money can usually buy you almost anything including a new identity and a fresh start.

Enrolment by abandonment is not common, but it does occasionally happen. In cases such as these, I try to look at the bright side. I like to think that we are a better place for the student than their actual home. Of course, this may not be true, but it has definitely proven true in the past, as in the case of Maria and now Max.

The gap between summer and regular school is usually one week, and Max was thrilled at the turn of events; he simply stayed in the same room he had been in all summer, although his room-mate had left when camp finished. Everyone leaves at the end of camp; even those who have decided to enrol for the regular school year. But Max simply turned up at the dining hall at meal times and was served, and went to bed at curfew time, just like he did during the summer. He even asked if he would be keeping the same room once school started.

As far as I'm aware, no one actually told him that his parents had abandoned him, although they did ask him if he had another number they could contact them on.

Max ended up being officially enrolled at school, and his parents were eventually reached. The excuses they made were the usual: travelling and not having their phones with them, or going to such far-flung places there was no internet or phone coverage, or simply claiming that the family 'secretary' had made a mistake and it was a simple misunderstanding.

Max spent the next three years at school and during that time I found out about his past. It turned out he had been a terrible bully, and had actually put a fellow student in hospital.

'I was an asshole,' is how he described his former self. I asked him what made him change. He said that he had been forced to go into hospital and see the damage he had done, made to apologise to his victim and the victim's family. 'You have no idea of the hurt you do.'

I can't remember Max getting into any trouble during the three years I knew him, although it did make me wonder what makes someone like Max become a bully. All I found out was that he was moved regularly, and had been raised by a fresh batch of strangers whenever he changed school.

I'm no psychologist but I do wonder if there was a sense of abandonment, much greater than the just being left behind after summer break, a sense of being alone in the world that was deep rooted in him, that made him make some bad decisions in his earlier years.

Thankfully, he learned from his mistakes early enough. He came out the other end a better person and a decent young man who, from this point on, will always try to be cool.

The Ivan effect

Part one

When I was a student, school trips consisted of hiking, more hiking, even more hiking, and hiking until we'd hiked so much we became lost in the woods. 'How much further?' everyone would grumble as we were led up a 2000-metre peak. We'd pitch our tents and wake up to fresh snow, a stream to be forded, and yet another peak to conquer. I loved every minute of it.

But things have changed since I was at school, and field trips are no longer designed to just be fun, they need to have an educational purpose. 'To experience other cultures,' we're often told, as students are sent to Rome, Barcelona, Paris or London.

Sure, these trips had the occasional trip-ups. Like the time I collected Federico from jail because he'd put a piece of the Coliseum in his backpack. 'It's just a bit of stone,' he'd said, protesting his innocence. Two hundred euros was enough to buy his freedom.

Then there was the time I had to pick up Denis from the secure room at the Galleria dell'Accademia in Florence after he was caught placing the wrapper of a chocolate bar in the hands of a convenient statue. He received a 100 euro fine. The money wasn't an issue, his family was incredibly wealthy – but his parents were suitably horrified when they found out. I stood by him when he made the phone call home. Awkward.

But it wasn't until a stay at a beautiful chateau in the south of France that I really felt I'd lost control. It was the annual Paris trip, which involved a quarter of the school spread out between homestays and hotels.

'It's the best time of year to go.' Marie was Head of the French Department and this was her tenth trip with the students. It was mid-spring and while it was still cool at night in the mountains, Marie kept reminding us that 'it's just right, not too hot or cold and no crowds'. This was my first time joining the trip. I figured the only way to get to grips with the French language was to immerse myself in it fully. I chaperoned Ivan and three other boys and we stayed in a bed and breakfast that was over half a century old.

I didn't know Ivan at all, but that's what's good about school trips; it's a chance to get along, and find out a bit about each other.

'You're supposed to be speaking French,' I snapped, during dinner. I was getting seriously peeved by Ivan's lack of manners. After asking the waiter if there was a McDonald's nearby, the boys had then asked to see a menu in English before simply ordering the same meals.

'I'm not good at French, and I'm hungry. Is that OK?' he retaliated.

It wasn't OK but it was the first night, so I kept the peace.

'So what are we to do tonight?' Ivan asked once he'd scoffed his fries and nuggets – not exactly your typical French cuisine, but they'd ordered from the children's menu. Dinner was over in twenty minutes and they were bored already.

'We must have some wine; that is French, yes?' Ivan was baiting me, but I enjoyed telling him no.

'But everyone else gets to drink, it's not fair.' The boys didn't have drinking permission as they were still one year shy of their senior year. It wasn't uncommon for students to be allowed one glass of wine on special trips, but it was entirely up to the person in charge.

I had planned an evening stroll through the village, and to meet up with a couple of the other groups, maybe wander into a bar and relax, but there was simply no way these likely lads were getting a drop while I was in charge.

It should have been magical walking through the cobbled streets of a medieval village, but the three of them were uninspired with such living history, and I was uninspired with them. At the earliest opportunity they retreated to their room and their gadgets.

Good night …

I was jolted awake at 3am by shouting coming from down the corridor, and I made my way to the boys' room.

I found the owner, our host, pleading for an answer from the boys.

'Why?' he begged. 'Just tell me why?'

The boys had destroyed the room. They'd burnt the towels and thrown them out the window. There were scorch marks on the wall, antique drawers, wardrobe, and the mirror was broken.

The pleading didn't move Ivan; he calmly opened his wallet and asked 'how much?'

The owner should have been raging, shaking his fists and lashing out at my boys, but he just wanted to know why. Ivan couldn't give him an answer, just a wallet full of cash.

'Get out, get out now, out …' spoke the owner deliberately, but Ivan didn't move.

'Calm down, we'll pay, just tell us how much … *combien*?'

Of all the opportunities he had had to use French, he had to start now.

'Out now or I'll call the police. You have five minutes.' This got through to Ivan and we all hurriedly packed our bags and made our escape.

'He overreacted, yeah?' Ivan was looking for the support of his friends, and they were unswerving in their loyalty.

'At least it's warm out tonight,' one of the lads said, at which point I was ready to explode. I could have physically strangled the lot of them.

The following Monday the boys were sent home for two weeks while the school decided if they would let them back. It was reassuring to know the parents were horrified – you never know what to expect from our parents. They readily paid for all the damage, and promised their sons would do whatever was necessary to stay at school. They even made donations.

Ivan was allowed back, but if he stepped out of line again, he'd be gone. If he failed his classes or talked back, he'd be gone. If he was caught smoking, drinking or even skipping class, he'd be gone. The school was ready to ban him from any further trips, but an exception was made …

Part two

'I'm not going.'

It was spring break and the students were going on a wide range of trips, many of which sounded fantastic: sailing, surfing, kayaking, even one that went to Scotland that involved golfing and a visit to a whisky distillery. But Ivan was going on a very different trip, to an orphanage in Lithuania. Although there were plenty of people wondering what the orphanage had done to deserve someone like Ivan.

Ivan was determined not to go to Lithuania, because, in his words, it was 'full of shitty poor people'. None of the teachers minded. Who would want him on such a trip, he'd only be a burden. But after a long discussion with his family, it was decided this particular excursion would do the troublemaker some good.

Ivan was going to spend a week living and working with children, from infants to teenagers, who were stricken by absolute poverty. How would someone like Ivan relate to someone who has nothing, not a single possession to call his or her own, not even parents?

Mr Driscoll once said there is no such thing as a bad child, just bad behaviour. I wanted this to be true, but at what age does your childhood leave you? I didn't care if Ivan was no longer a child, he was eighteen years old and legally an adult, I simply wanted to see if he had the ability to show compassion and empathy towards other human beings. Ivan and I were to be travelling buddies once more.

Would he let me down again?

Ivan made a friend on the first day of the trip, even though he wasn't looking for one. Anastasia climbed into his lap. She was six years old and all she knew was the orphanage.

'She likes you,' said our host, a middle-aged woman who had spent her entire life looking after the poor. Ivan didn't know how to react, but Anastasia did.

'What's your name?' she asked, as she pulled his arms around her. Ivan mumbled a reply.

After this, Anastasia was permanently attached to Ivan. She pulled him around the orphanage showing him where she ate, slept and played.

Everyone in the group made friends with the children. The workers at the orphanage were female and they kept on reminding us that most of their children had never had an older male influence in their lives.

It's not possible to be human and not show compassion when confronted by such realities.

'They seem so happy,' I remember Ivan saying. He'd been there two days and thanks to Anastasia I was beginning to see a different side of him. And he was right, they did seem happy. 'But they have nothing,' he added, sounding perplexed.

They didn't even have a proper football because the one they'd been using for years was patched over and kept on deflating. When Ivan bought them a new ball, he was swamped with hugs from the youngest orphans, while the older teenagers got competitive and enjoyed thrashing the visitors in a friendly game. I couldn't believe how such a small gift could be so appreciated.

After that, everyone started buying gifts. It's what we can do to help. A new cot, new blankets, new sporting equipment, even a laptop, although the internet wasn't the most reliable. But what meant even more to the orphans was people spending time with them, even if our lot didn't always have a choice in the matter. When the students sat down, a small child would make their way to a spare knee or lap; Ivan's lap belonged to Anastasia.

'They don't have much physical contact,' explained Greta, the woman in charge. 'People don't want to hug them, especially someone with HIV.' Some of the kids are HIV positive, she had explained, but thanks to the UN and WHO they got their medicines for free.

On the morning of our departure Ivan was in tears. He was saying farewell to Anastasia who had her own trickle of water down her cheeks. How does one say goodbye in situations like this? You know you'll never see them again, and as you go back to your secure world, you realise such things don't exist for these children, and you suddenly appreciate just what you have.

That week changed Ivan forever.

In my opinion, all students should be made to go on humanitarian trips just like this. As educators, I feel it is our duty to educate not just the mind, but the soul.

Fun in the sun

Not all trips abroad are life changing. Admittedly, I often volunteer to be a 'responsible adult' on a trip simply because it sounds like so much fun; sometimes I even get to plan my own trip.

Strangely enough I've discovered that I'm quite good at arranging these, especially when it's the students who are paying. The senior Greek sailing trip was a particularly inspired idea, or so I thought.

'You don't know what you're missing, Mohammed.' We were sitting on the deck of the yacht while I was regaling everyone with memories from my school days. 'You can't beat roughing it in the bush,' I said. There was a collective groan and rolling of eyes.

'But we are roughing it,' Mohammed said. 'Abdullah hasn't had a shower in two days.' There were some chuckles at Mohammed's remark. 'I thought the yachts would be a bit bigger. I feel I've been deceived,' he added.

For the last two nights we'd slept out at sea, cooked our own food, learned a bit about sailing, had our first scuba diving lesson, and despite the occasional attempt at complaining about the cramped quarters, everyone was having an absolute blast. But now we were headed to a popular island famous for its night life.

We were trailed by a second yacht, the girls' yacht, led by the trip leader, Johnno.

The students had been pleading for some free time at a local night spot on one of the islands. 'We're seniors. It's my last year at school. I want to have some fun,' Mohammed said. Mohammed had argued his case many times in the last 48 hours. It was an argument the rest of the group echoed incessantly. 'We do have drinking permission. Other seniors on other trips get to drink.'

'You don't even drink alcohol. It's against your religion for crying out loud.'

'But I like to buy my friends a drink,' he replied.

Johnno and I had agreed on a compromise. Once we set foot on land, we were going to have a traditional dinner together at a restaurant recommended by our captains, and allow the kids some wine with their meal. 'It wouldn't be traditional without a shot of Ouzo,' complained Nikita. We ignored his remark.

The food was superb, the wine adequate, and the boys were enjoying spending an evening together with the girls. The only problem with the meal wasn't the food itself, but the loud music blaring out of a local bar just down the road.

'Maybe we should check it out.'

'We can't sleep with such a racket.'

'It would be culturally insensitive not to go to a local club.'

'Greece is the land of sun, sand and se—' I cut Joel off before he could finish his sentence, but the girls were already giggling.

'I think that glass of wine has affected you already.' Joel scoffed at such a suggestion.

Reluctantly we made our way back to the docked yachts.

'Well, this isn't fair.'

'Tell them to be quiet.'

'This is torture.'

The yachts were moored directly opposite the noisy nightclub. Instead of getting ready for bed, everyone was sitting on the side of the yacht looking forlornly at the people going in and out of the bar. In the dimly lit night you could make out the silhouettes of people dancing through the open windows.

'This is truly cruel, sir,' Mohammed said to me, and I had to agree with him. Johnno and I made an executive decision. 'Well, I suppose it would be all right, if we went with you.' There were cheers all round. 'But ... you are to be on your best behaviour. One drink only per person, and when we say it's time to leave, we leave, no argument.'

'Thank you so much, sir. The first round is on me,' Mohammed offered.

'You mean the only round,' I replied.

'Yes, that's what I meant.'

To our surprise there was a door charge to get in, but without hesitation Mohammed paid for everyone, and true to his word he also paid for everyone's drinks.

His generosity impressed everyone, creating an atmosphere of good fun and good will. Mohammed found himself a couch near the wall where he could watch the room. His fellow Saudis stayed with him while the girls went off to dance with the rest of the boys.

'There's something strange about this place,' Johnno observed. We'd been there about twenty minutes and I had to agree; something didn't seem quite right. We'd been so busy making sure the kids got in OK and had only one drink each, we hadn't paid much attention to the rest of the setting.

We noticed a local looking man had pulled up a chair and was sitting with Mohammed and the gang. Johnno and I sidled into the background, within hearing distance, just in case he was up to no good.

The man offered to buy Mohammed and his friends some drinks, but they politely refused. He then tried some small talk; he asked the guys where they were from, and offered them a cigarette each. Our boys turned down his offer, but did say they were from Saudi Arabia. Johnno and I were on guard, and I could sense Mohammed becoming wary too, but before we had a chance to intervene, the stranger made his move.

Men and women do it to each other all the time; a brief touch, a false smile, a forced laugh. The first point of contact seemed almost innocuous, as he rocked back and forth at some great jest, his hand landing on Mohammed's knee as if driven by the force of so much hilarity.

'Did you see that? I don't believe it. Did you see it?' Johnno exclaimed. I had seen it. Mohammed looked in our direction, a stricken look on his face. We returned his look of distress with a smile and a wave. 'I think we should do something. This could get nasty,' I said.

'You're right, but that was truly priceless.'

As we approached them, we could see Mohammed's look of terror as he sat staring at the stranger's hand still upon his knee.

'You look so strong, so …' The stranger never got a chance to finish as Johnno and I pulled up chairs opposite and, catching the hint, the man wandered away.

'Did you see that? What the fuck was that?' Mohammed and the other Saudis were quite worked up. 'He put his hand on my knee.'

'He obviously liked you.' The boys didn't know how to react. They tried to look indignant and unruffled at the same time.

I asked Mohammed why he was so eager to pay for everyone to go to a gay bar.

'What the … I didn't want this …'

'You paid for everyone,' I reminded him.

His mouth dropped. 'I'm in a gay bar? My father can never find out about this.'

We chose that moment to call it a night. We'd only been there an hour, but the group kept their word and didn't complain.

'Hey guys, Mohammed took us to a gay bar,' Johnno called out when we'd regrouped. Eventually Mohammed and his friends saw the funny side, although they never found it as hilarious as the rest of us!

EPILOGUE

Graduation

I'm not one of 'them', but they need people like me.

I'm not super rich, or even mildly rich; I've never had servants or bodyguards; I've never driven a Porsche or Ferrari let alone owned one, and I wouldn't know how to behave at the high society functions and fundraisers their parents throw. It's exactly for this reason they need me, not as a nurse, but as a regular guy.

These kids need a whole lot of 'regular' guys, whether they, or their parents, realise it ...

Mr Fitzpatrick was the head of the most exclusive and expensive school around, a whopping 140,000 euros a year for tuition and board, and I was part of a group that were being given a tour of his campus. I was mingling with board members, headmasters and recruiters. We all knew I didn't belong; I was only there to check out the health centre.

The campus was, as you'd expect, outstanding, yet the most poignant memory for me was when someone asked how they could justify such an incredible price.

'It's an expensive country,' he began, 'and that's what parents like about it. A lot of our parents don't want their child mingling with common people and such a high price ensures this.' Such words should have been spoken as a confession, instead he sounded proud.

There are over 7000 international schools around the world, with more than three million students, and the forecast is for that number to double in the next ten years. That's a lot of teachers (around 300,000) and a lot of nurses; and it's us regular guys who have a responsibility to bring out the compassion and humanity that resides in these kids as well as in all of us.

I'm optimistic that not all wealthy parents are as Mr Fitzpatrick described, and I know that the vast majority of the students do care, but with so many future leaders in the making, whether business, technology, politics or other positions of power, we need the kids to understand and value the common man.

There are other reasons why parents spend a lot of money to send their child to a boarding school like ours:

Safety. For some, this is the only time when the students won't have a driver or bodyguard. One year there was a surge in kidnappings in Mexico and Brazil, and our numbers from those parts doubled.

Networking. When you spend as much as nine to ten years living, growing, experimenting, playing and learning with someone, you have a friend for life whom you can trust. I suspect knowing who to trust is not easy for some, especially when inheriting wealth or power.

Prestige. For the parents, not so much the kids.

Work. Some schools began as a place for children of ex-pats working in corners of the world that are dangerous or undeveloped. Often the companies they work for pay for their children's schooling abroad.

Effort. Sadly, some parents just don't want to deal with their children; it's sometimes hard to see it as neglect when parents spend so much money.

And my favourite:

Scholarships. Sometimes the regular guys make it in.

Some schools are required by law to take a certain number of scholarship students, and while some take the minimum number, others take more. Almost without fail, it's the scholarship students who do the best. They appreciate the value of their education, and many come from hardship, even poverty.

Many teachers tell me they like having these students in class as they set a good example, though the others don't always follow.

It makes sense that those with nothing strive to do better, although it makes me wonder how those who've had everything can appreciate what they have.

Many of our students don't. It's not their fault, and they're not bad kids, they just don't know about the real world. School headmasters, those like Mr Fitzpatrick, should make it their goal to admit as many 'common' people as possible. But ultimately private education is a business, and while we can educate the children, we can't enlighten the parents.

But once a year, I get an opportunity to try …

The grand finale

'It's a beautiful prison,' Andrew joked, but he still looked close to shedding a tear. The two of us were standing outside the Grand Hall, waiting for the parents to settle down and the ceremony to begin.

Andrew had spent his life in boarding school, well, at least the important parts of his life so far. He had spent his formative years here, those years when your body begins to change and you discover that the opposite sex is much more fun than your favourite stuffed toy.

'You'll never all be together in the same place again,' I added poignantly.

'Thanks, that really helps.' But he couldn't help but smile at my lack of tact. 'I'll never see this place again,' he added and I told him how wrong he was.

The long-termers always come back, at least once, no matter how far and wide they spread and they spread pretty far: from the Arctic circle to the tail of New Zealand, from the Steppes of Kazakhstan to the rain forests of Brazil.

'Nah, I'm done. I'll miss my friends, but I need to get off this mountain.'

'You'll be back … and I'll probably still be here!' I said, unsure of whether I was joking.

'I hope so, you're one of the good guys.'

Dammit, he was going to get me all soppy with such talk. Graduation days stir up mixed emotions, happiness and sadness. I've been there during the good times and bad, the breaks, the triumphs, the tragedies. They're kids no more, they're young adults who've turned out, for the most part, pretty damn fine. The road hasn't always been easy, and there's been blood, sweat and tears shed, but they made it. And I made it as well.

Andrew filed into the Grand Hall and officially finished high school.

The Grand ceremony in the Grand Hall is followed by a Grand Dinner, with families and staff mingling. It's my chance to meet, and hopefully not confront, the people who've sometimes ordered, yelled, and sometimes even thanked me, over the phone.

Over the past ten graduations I've attended, I've met the parents of nearly all the special characters who have come into my life.

When Ameena graduated, her parents were lovely, rational, and seemingly incapable of hate, although I never did find out if they ever discovered their daughter's friendship with a Jewish girl. And had it actually mattered?

When Kurt's mother asked me how her son got the scar on his forehead, Kurt gave me a very worried stare. I resisted the urge to say: 'If you think that's bad, you ought to check out his fore …'

When Faisal, the Lebanese rocket launching warrior graduated, he and his parents shook hands with all his teachers, even the Jewish ones. I often joke that I only go to graduation for the food, and to ogle the cars in the parking lot, but I'm just kidding. For me, graduation is a chance for the young adults and staff to say farewell.

Perhaps I too will graduate soon. I don't know how much longer I'll stay a school nurse, because I feel a touch of guilt. Sure, I have a lot of responsibility and I do make a difference, and I do enjoy working with children, but I want to make a greater difference, change the lives of the poor, not just the rich.

Whether this means going to a developing nation and working with those most in need, or simply returning to New Zealand and doing some good close to home, I'm not so sure. I'll guess I'll just have to wait and see …

Acknowledgements

Again, how do you thank the people who made you what you are? From friends, family, patients and colleagues, you have all had an impact on my life, in work and home, in fun times and sad, and this book would not have been possible without you.

I would also like to thank Rachel from The Friday Project for being so patient and working so hard.

Thanks everyone.